Advance Praise for *Where's My Crown for Acting Like Everything Is Fine?*

"Kerstin's writing draws you in and makes you feel like you're sitting on the couch with an old friend for wine night. We are all waiting for something. Whether it's big and exciting or small and mundane, Kerstin reminds us to not focus so much on what we're waiting for or we might miss what's right in front of us. And even though the waiting can feel heavy and painful, there is always joy and hope to be found in the present. Thank you, Kerstin for reminding us that we are all so much more alike than we are different and to embrace each moment we've been given."

—Corie Clark, Creator of the Purposeful Planner, Author, Educator, Blogger on CorieClark.com

"A must read! Spiritually uplifting, remarkably inciteful, with just the right splash of humor, Lindquist's book provides a feeling of comfort that reaches deep inside us. Waiting for the rug to be pulled out from under us is exhausting, but Kerstin guides us to trust in the Lord's Word, which she richly provides in her book. Through prayer we are reassured that He will show us the way to relaxation and happiness. No one is

perfect. Perfection is perception, and we need to look to God to help us perceive what we are meant to be, to help us grab our crown!"

—Kate Redeker, Miss Wisconsin USA 2016

"What you are waiting for might be found in this book, maybe. Or it could be lost running from a very hectic life, insisting... 'Everything is fine!' Kerstin Lindquist has done it again! Given reason to fall into grace, love beyond fear and thrive in the wisdom of the great waiting rooms of life. Practicality and hope for those moments when you're wondering, 'when will things get better?' This work is a crowning achievement, teaching the very fundamentals in giving and receiving love for self, community and the Divine."

—J.R. Mahon, Spiritual Director &
Executive Director of TableTop Ministries

"It is to me like sitting having a hot cup of tea with my best friend who would never lie to me. Straight talk and heartfelt; warm and comforting. Wonderful reminders of everything we should be doing every day. Excellent examples of how we should do as Jesus did, not live our lives as we perceive others see us. A lot of relatable life experiences and an easy read. You forget that others often have gone through what you have or that you maybe are the one to guide others through their valleys."

—Trish Redeker, Mom, wife, empty nester

"Kerstin's writing is powerful. Her personal testimonies teach us how to thrive in life's many waiting periods. She offers practical tips that will not only inspire you, but also bring comfort and peace in the midst of your waiting."

—Roma Downey, Emmy
Nominated Actress, Producer,
and *New York Times* Bestselling Author

"I could not put this book down. Kerstin has a way with words that makes you just keep going to the next page! She calls you to be your best self, despite the reality that for most of life we are stuck in a waiting room, caught between the now and the not yet. I love her insights on the bestselling book of Esther, a true story of a woman much like us! Kerstin will inspire you to wake up early, put on your best workout clothes, and move! She will brainwash you to like foods that you thought you'd never like, and motivate you to wear that crown that you were always meant to wear, all with childlike wonder and eyes on eternity."

—Monica Guaglione, Director
of Education, Innovative Academy
Calvary Chapel Chadds Ford

WHERE'S MY CROWN FOR ACTING LIKE EVERYTHING IS FINE?

ROYALLY SURVIVING LIFE'S WAITING PERIODS

KERSTIN LINDQUIST

POST HILL PRESS

A POST HILL PRESS BOOK
ISBN: 978-1-64293-485-4
ISBN (eBook): 978-1-64293-486-1

Where's My Crown for Acting Like Everything Is Fine?:
Royally Surviving Life's Waiting Periods
© 2020 by Kerstin Lindquist
All Rights Reserved

Cover photo by Scott C. Kinkade
Author portrait courtesy of Perscky Photography

This is a work of nonfiction. All people, locations, events, and situations are portrayed to the best of the author's memory.

Post Hill Press
New York • Nashville
posthillpress.com

Published in the United States of America

CONTENTS

INTRODUCTION: FINE

"Fine. I'm fine. We're all fine."

That's the qualifying phrase that always seems to follow the list of things that are anything but fine. Why do we do that? You're not fine. We aren't fine. Nothing seems to be fine! It's hard. Life is hard. But we seem to do a *fine* job of convincing everyone around us, including ourselves, that everything is just fine.

Stop. Just stop. It's okay to not be okay.

We've been taught since Sunday school that this time on earth isn't the real deal. The party begins when we get to heaven. Everyone we lost will be found. Those relationships that were cut short by illness and age will be restored. There will be abundant beauty and calm and all the wine and cheese without any of the regrets. No wonder we can't wait to get there. No wonder we wish away time. Heaven sounds a whole lot easier than what we're dealing with back on earth. But not so fast, there is a lot of living left to do here first.

It's just sometimes that living part is so hard. It can seem nearly unbearable to survive, let alone thrive in the meantime.

Great word: *mean*time. Life isn't easy; it can be so mean. And while we're waiting, we can be pretty mean to ourselves. Living in what often seems like a cruel world doesn't have to translate to ignoring what's happening around us in the name of just getting to heaven. And it sure doesn't mean pretending everything is great. It's not. And we've got work to do. It's why God put us here in the first place. The Lord gave you those skills, that job, this family, those struggles for some purpose. The discovery then becomes a waiting of its own. It could be big: waiting for a partner with whom to navigate this life, waiting for a child to complete your family, waiting for the cancer to be gone. Or it could be less momentous: like waiting for clarity on a decision, waiting for the promotion, or waiting for a rough season to pass. It could be the daily wait: waiting in line, waiting for the kids to stop screaming, or waiting to get a freaking break! We are all waiting on something, and waiting is not easy.

We need to consider that those waiting rooms of life that we so dread are full of gifts we're just too frustrated to find. Maybe you aren't getting out because there is something in there you are meant to discover. A person, a place, a situation that will change your life, or theirs, for the better. You just need to stop trying so hard to find the door that leads out. This waiting room is right where you're supposed to be.

In the days you spend with this book you are going to learn to survive this wait. And every wait that life brings you after this one. Because, dear one, it never ends. Don't groan that sentence away like I know you will. If you can learn to find happiness and joy and fulfillment in these waiting periods of life you will be better prepared, or dare I say, even excited about the next one to come. That's what you will learn in these pages. Each wait is different and each one has a story. I will share some of the hardest waiting periods of my life and I pray this will teach you to share yours. We aren't rushing to get through these times, pretending we're okay. We are sitting in them and looking around us and allowing our grief to be a piece of the learning. I pray you will find inspiration whether you have been waiting five days or five years.

——————✧——————

For most of my adult life I haven't been able to quit a book. I never jumped to the end to see what happened, and I never, ever stopped reading a book early, no matter how unsatisfactory I found it. My husband finally convinced me that my time was worth more than a bad read. If I didn't like it, I'd skip to the end to see what the outcome was and then move on. While I still feel guilty at times, this practice of skipping over what isn't bringing me joy has been a huge breakthrough. Here's what I'm giving you—the end. You will come out of this stronger, better prepared, and hopefully, happier as you move into the next wait. You will learn to be authentic and honest with yourself and those around you. But you need to do the work. At the end of each chapter you will be given action, as well as practices and tools that will help you move through this season.

Six areas of focus:

1. Protecting your mind.
2. Getting fit for the fight.
3. Sharing your story.
4. Finding your support.
5. Resting.
6. Accepting God's timing.

This is a time of growth. It's scary and many of you might be in tremendous pain in this wait. Oh, sister, how my heart hurts for you. I don't know you personally, but I *do* know you because I have been there. Broken, bruised, afraid I would never come up for air. I promise there is hope. This wait isn't going to break you. This life isn't too much, even though it so often feels that way. You will come out stronger and you will survive even if the worst-case scenario becomes reality. Once you learn to straighten your crown and waltz your way through this wait, you can finally move on, because each waiting room leads to the next, until we eventually get to the place we are all waiting for: home, on our throne, with our heavenly father.

"Yet the Lord longs to be gracious to you;
therefore he will rise up to show you compassion.
For the Lord is a God of justice.
*Blessed are all who **wait** for him!"*
(Isaiah 30:18 NIV)

PROTECT YOUR MIND

When my thoughts tend to go to *what if?*
Lead me back to *but God.*

1

OLD WOMAN IN THE SHOE

have an actor friend; let's call him Jason because this is not a book about giving away celebrity secrets. Movies and television have been his job for over twenty years. He's not often in the pages of gossip magazines and pop culture news programs, but I bet you would recognize him if you passed him on the street, or at least take a second look. He has a presence. You just know he's *someone*. He's one of the people in my life whom I consider a part of my spiritual support group—something so important for you to have in these times of waiting. Each time we talk, whether it's about our kids, or work, or really good food (this guy crushes food; seriously, his metabolism is quite admirable) we don't get more than a few words in without mentioning our walk with the Lord. It may be something that came up in morning prayer, or a podcast we heard, or what God's doing in our lives and the lives of our families, but God is always in the discussion. It's one of my favorite relationships because of this fact. We've seen each other through divorce, job loss, marriage, births, and everything in-between. God has been right there in all of it with us, and has used my friendship with this man (who can eat a dozen donuts after breakfast and not put on a pound, honestly, he is a superhero) to teach me so much.

Despite so many parallels in our professions, it's hard for me to stomach what he does. He never knows where his next paycheck is coming from. He is constantly hustling and auditioning and trusting every day that the next day will bring rewards. He has forever been dependent like a child on the Lord's provision. There were times when rent was past due, and he had to put his faith in his father to provide. Month after month, year after year. There have been years of plenty and overflow but there have been even more seasons of scarcity and drought. He always trusts. His is a life of constant wait, but he always trusts.

I, on the other hand, am always waiting for the other shoe to drop. My trust in life is lacking. Pray? Yes. Rely on God? Of course. But trust it will all be okay? Not a chance. Is that being a woman, a mom, a control freak? Ha. Yes, all three, I'm sure. There have been many times in my life when the wait was inconsequential—waiting for winter to end, waiting for sales to pick up, waiting for a child to be potty trained. The waiting room I was in was actually quite peaceful and packed with contentment. But what I really felt I was waiting for in those times was for the big bad thing to happen again.

The big, bad thing.

Would it be cancer, or job loss, or black mold? With such a blessed, full life, I always feel so vulnerable to loss. Because my waits have been traumatic, I never fully trust that this good life is here to stay. What is the next thing I will need to tackle? What will steal my joy?

Here is where I say, *stop being like me and waiting for the bad. Live in the good. Don't put that negativity into the universe.* But that is not what I'm going to write. Because something does always seem to happen. An event occurs, an email arrives, the results come back and just like that all the shoes from flip flops to cowboy boots come crashing into that peaceful room in which you've been waiting. The difference between me and Jason is that he accepts this as life. He expects God will show up and hold his hand through the hard. He lives in the shoe drop. I try to put that ugly shoe back in the box and return it. Nope, not for me thank you very much, I'd like my money back.

While it's healthy to expect the best, it is irrational to have an expectation of constant ease. There is an important distinction here. Expecting the best doesn't mean you have unrealistic expectations. Jason isn't expecting everything will be perfect and easy even in times of plenty, but he is believing that no matter what happens God will be there to get him through it. Ahhh, yes, there you see. Expectations from God are different from expectations from this world.

Expecting the best doesn't mean you have unrealistic expectations.

There are many coaches I follow and books I read and conferences I attend that keep me striving for my best life. This wisdom comes in the form of mantras and journaling and goal setting. Girl, I am all about all of that! If I could, I would go from conference to workshop professionally. I thrive on positive input and daily encouragement. You should see my planner; it is awash in verses and phrases that keep me present and peaceful. I do a morning devotional that includes listing what I'm grateful for and my daily goals, as well as long-term plans. Every Sunday I look back on the week and list my accomplishments and set new goals for the week. I truly believe in all of this positive thinking and strategic planning.

But, that's not enough. It's just not.

No amount of planning and goal-setting is going to keep life from happening. This is me trying to control the outcome of an uncontrollable world. In fact, control isn't even a biblical word. We can say, *I give God control*, but that isn't meaningful to our Lord. There is no control. He wants us to depend on Him through the chaos, because that is life. No one is in control; we can only change our responses.

Then what do we do, crazy lady, with the control complex and colorful day planner? Glad you asked. You live in the shoe drop. But you don't live there alone. As with every conversation I've had in nearly ten years with Jason, you do it with God in the middle. No matter what shoe drops, imagine your Lord right there next to you, fitting you for the next size up. Put on all those shoes that seem to rain from heaven and wear them like a boss.

Live in the shoe drop.

Now work on what you expect from Him. You can absolutely assume the Lord's help in getting you to the next chapter, but as soon as you allow your expectation of an easy path to take over your thought life—become the things you dwell on and dream about—you will be set up for disappointment. That doesn't mean you don't plan and pray and expect joy. But joy can come even in the pain. That is the ultimate goal. Joy in all this pain. Yes, we are good people, smart people, women who love the Lord and serve our families and others and pay our taxes and hold the door open and smile at everyone. But bad things are still going to happen. It's not fair, but as we have all learned, life isn't fair. Stay with me here; we need to be thankful for every difficult outcome because it is getting us closer to our God. We turn around and lean into Him and He gives us back the strength to keep going and be stronger for the next hurdle. Because the next waiting room is just down the hall. Yep, come this way. Another wait, aren't you stoked?

Sweet child, imagine living your life like a six-five Hollywood leading man that can eat anything he wants. Be Jason. Eat the cake and trust in God (how's that for a bumper sticker?). Where I want you to be is in that place where you have zero expectation of what is next. You are living in the moment and reacting to what God is giving you right now. When the days are blissful and all is right with the world, I want you—*He wants you*—to soak that in and pour out your songs of gratitude for the blessings He has provided. Dive into His word and read all you can. Get out there and serve others in their loss. When people ask how you are doing, really tell them how great you are and give the credit to God. Experience that high. You deserve it. Please don't hide that light for fear of it being extinguished by the reactions of others. Don't constantly expect the bad thing to happen at dawn, but also don't expect that struggles won't arise. And when the shoe drops, take those reserves and use them. Lean into the Lord and expect He will hold your hand or even carry you through. This isn't struggling, this is living!

And you are right now, in this book, in this chapter of your life, acquiring the tools to find the good in every shoe that drops.

———————✧———————

Don't Wait:

- When you are in a place of plenty, prepare for the coming winter. There are many seasons and in the good ones we need to read and pray and study to ready our hearts and minds and even our bodies for what's to come. Find another good book. Journal. Please, for the love of little baby Jesus, read the bible! It's amazing how simple it really is. Read. The. Bible. His answers and instructions are all right there.
- When the other shoe does drop, live in it. Accept this time as a part of living and find the joy in the pain. Allow yourself to grieve; that's an important part of your healing. But don't let your dashed expectations define the moment.
- Don't be a slave to your emotions but witness them and then turn to the Lord. Give them to the Lord so he can fill you back up with Him instead of exhaustive despair.
- Release your expectations of the world and what it owes you, and instead expect your Lord to be there for you, no matter what the world throws at you.

———————✧———————

I have been in a period of major transition for what feels like forever; illness, loss of my parents, moves, career change, all in the last five years. I spent most of my time asking God why and when will it get better? I have now figured out that this period of waiting, while excruciatingly difficult was not only necessary in making me stronger but a part of His plan all along. This realization doesn't make the process any easier, as I'm not the most patient person, but I take comfort in knowing there is purpose in the pain and that something new is beginning. I'm waiting for restoration and my new beginning.

—Brooke

2

SUCH A TIME AS THIS

When we first moved east from California, I looked on a map and found the closest beach to our new landlocked home. I was a Cali girl, born and raised, and I couldn't quite wrap my head around living so far from the ocean. That first summer I would pack up my two two-year-olds and drive the hour and a half to the bay for even a few hours of water time. Two-year-olds in the car are an interesting exercise in stress management. I didn't just have one to deal with, I had two. I happened to be doing a Beth Moore study on James at the time, and she challenged us to memorize the book. I don't know what made me think I had the time, patience, or even mental capacity as a mom of toddlers working full-time shift work, but I printed out the first few verses and gave it a go. I would recite the words over and over again in my head aloud as I drove the hour back and forth from the beach, week after week. Between crying babies, traffic, and the oppressive east coast heat this California beach girl was not prepared for, I would recite "count it all joy," and "remember the testing of your faith" was going to "produce endurance." Endurance, I needed endurance for sure.

I did it. I memorized the entire book in a few months. Now don't be too impressed, James is a short book, a baby book, but each verse is packed with such rich goodness. That book changed my life. We throw that phrase around a little too much; *that show changed my life, that hair dryer changed my life, that meal changed my life!* But in the case of James, it's true. My life has been exponentially enhanced by memorizing scripture. It's amazing how, from that crazy summer forward, the Lord has poured those words from my mouth at the perfect times. When I have nothing to give a friend in need or a sister in crisis, these verses just flow. For me, when the anxiety builds, and my mind starts racing, I instantly recall, "blessed is a man who perseveres under pressure" (James 1:12 NIV) or "for we all stumble in many ways," (James 3:2 NIV) and the repetition results in release. When I question what I'm doing with my life and if I'm really hearing the Lord, I repeat James 2:18: "I will show you my faith by my works."

That summer started my yearning for verse memorization. I fervently studied and consumed verses on fear and pain and love and trials. It has since grown to include not just verses but phrases, sayings, words I read in books. It doesn't matter really where the lines come from, but the act of memorization is key here. It's meditative, gets me out of my own head. And it's amazing how these thoughts will come back when I need them most. They all swim in and out at any given time. They don't all stay put. Now, years after I memorized James, I can't recite the entire book on cue, but it's still there at God's disposal. He pours it out of me when He needs.

Which leads me to such a time as this. The verse I cherish more than any other: "…and who knows but that you have come to your royal position for such a time as this?" (Esther 4:14 NIV) Of all the verses and quotes that I've spent time on, only two have meant enough to me that I've contemplated tattooing them on my body. I haven't, yet, but don't put it past me. Esther 4:14 has taken me through death and yearning and pain and fear. I consider Esther one badass chick who I would love to meet. When that question about who you would want at dinner, living or dead, comes around, Esther is top five. Her and Ruth. If you're significant enough to be the only two women in the most famous book of all time, to have a chapter named after you, then I want to have dinner…and drinks…maybe a spring retreat.

I don't even remember how I really came upon Esther 4:14. I did an Esther study and had read that story numerous times before I zeroed in on the significance of the passage. Now I have the framed picture of these words on my wall, and the phrase scribbled on nearly every page of my daily planner. They paraphrase this most popular verse in the book of Esther. The one I memorized and live out every day reads: "…*perhaps this is the moment for what you have been created.*" Yet, when you read the book what you find is actually: "…*and who knows but that you have come to your royal position for such a time as this?*" (Esther 4:14 NIV)

The most popular verse, in one of only two female-focused books in the number one best seller in all humanity takes us into a biblical waiting room.

Wow. Maybe we need to give that some love.

Now granted, we have that royal situation to account for, and chances are, like me, you aren't Meghan Markle, but we'll look past that for a moment. Let's trust in the scholars and live in *such a time as this.*

Your time. Right now. This struggle. This wait. It's big and it's yours.

And you know what? It's not going to end and miraculously everything will be perfect. That's not how it works. "There is no there, there,"[1] as Gertrude Stein wrote, and Shauna Niequist so eloquently restated in her book *Present Over Perfect*. We can't let all our happiness depend on getting to the end of this struggle. Once you get there, there is another struggle brewing. One waiting room leads to the next, and the next and the next, each one having its own time and purpose.

Yes, there is a purpose, which is why it is so important to be present in *this* time. I know this all sounds exhausting, the constant jump from one wait to the next. It can feel endless and hopeless and can easily send you to the couch with a pint of ice cream and hours of Netflix. But it doesn't have to. If you let the reality of the harshness of life take over your brain space, of course you will want to shut down, but if you take back your thought life and meditate on the good and the present, you will find joy in each new space. Philippians 4:8 says exactly this: "...whatever is true, whatever is noble, whatever is right, whatever is pure, whatever is lovely, whatever is admirable—if anything is excellent or praiseworthy—think about such things."

Think about such things. Good things. Powerful things. Things full of hope and joy and happiness. Things that make you smile. This may be hard right now; there may be very little that brings you joy. Perhaps you can't even remember the last time your eyes lit up.

---

[1] page 298 of Gertrude Stein's *Everybody's Autobiography*, published in 1937

That's why memorization can be a huge tool. Find what is good and dwell on it by repeating it over and over. Go to the bible, a book, social media if that helps. (Though that can be a slippery slope. In a time like this, everyone's joy can make things seem even worse, so be careful.) Start filling up with the good. Memorize, study, repeat.

This is a battle my friend. A battle for your mind.

When I was finally pregnant with my middle child—the miracle baby, as she likes to call herself (insert eye roll here), the only biological and the only one that ever stuck around long enough to be born alive—I had a high-risk OBGYN who repeatedly told me to "protect your mind." I hated being pregnant because a) I was not a happy human maker; I was a hot mess the entire time, and b) I was scared to death. From the time they implanted her, through the two-weeks wait, through every progesterone suppository and the endless blood tests, even when I had gained sixty pregnancy pounds and I felt two hundred months pregnant and wanted her out more than anything, I was still scared I would lose her. I'd had too many miscarriages and failed fertility treatments and every day I thought would bring another loss. This was a nine-month waiting period that, funnily, has now turned into an eighteen-year waiting period where I am still petrified of what could happen to her. You see, it never ends. Lord have mercy. You need to guard your mind in the process, because our thoughts have such awesome power. My doctor couldn't promise me a happy outcome this time around. But he could help me focus on the now—the beauty (wrong word, I was less than beautiful at eight months huge, but go with it) of being pregnant in that moment. Such a time as this.

Don't Wait:

- Memorize the passage. I've spent countless months on countless bible studies that challenge you to memorize passages, but "only if you have the time." "Only if you really want to." I'm not here to let you off the hook. If you are reading this, you have a desire to improve something in your life, to develop tools that will allow you to thrive in the place you are no matter how in the weeds you feel. So, I'm telling you: memorize. Meditate on the good. I recommend Esther 4:14 to start. We're talking at most an hour of your life to cement it into your subconscious. You can give that to God, and you can give that to yourself. Write it down, type it out on a note in your phone, scribble it on a piece of paper and put it in your calendar, and then say it over and over and over. It brings such calm in chaos. Pick your translation, or use the paraphrase that has gotten me through, but just do it.
- From there, keep going. Expand the good words in your mind. I have a verse or mantra, one for when I give a talk or go on air: "Let the words of my mouth and the meditation of my heart be acceptable to you." I have one for before I sit down to study the word: "Fill me up so that I may pour out." And there can be so much more. List the top five situations in a day that bring you to a boiling point and find meditative words for that situation that can help you refocus. I've listed verses and phrases in the memorization section at the end of this book that can help you find the words you're looking for.

- Read Esther 4. She was in a waiting period beyond anything any of us could imagine. In order to save the Jews from slaughter, she had to risk her own execution. Talk about being in your head and full of anxiety and worry. Yet this decision and this wait was not about her. God was using her in this situation, and her faithfulness to Him is what would get her and her people through this time. You may be in a spot in your life where you must have the courage and faithfulness to trust God to see it through. We are not called to rely on ourselves, ever, but on our Lord. "I know Lord that a person's way of life is not his own. No one who walks determines his own steps." (Jer.10:23)

- Esther accepted the challenge, but she would not go talk to the king on her own. She called on the Lord through prayer and fasting. What do you need to be on your knees in prayer for right now? What can you fast from, be it food or technology or something else that demands your attention? Try giving it up for this next week, and when it comes to mind, direct that energy to prayer. As an ease into fasting from food, stop eating by six or seven at night and don't eat again until nine the next morning, spend that morning in prayer focused on such a time as this.

———✤———

When my husband was sent to prison for three years, I was in shock. Alone, confused, angry, questioning everything, losing faith and not understanding why. We had a newborn, he had been clean and sober for six months, I waited for this happiness and family and now it was ripped away. Sixteen months into my wait for him, I am learning. I know my greatness has not yet begun fully. There is more to come. And every time I look into my son's big blue eyes and he smiles back at me the fear and anxiety stop and I remember to be present in this blessed time.

—Diana

3

POCKETS OF HAPPY

Been in the weeds for about a week. Funky with all the stuff. But had to share a pocket of happy.

Just realized I'm naked in my kitchen making myself a martini. 😂

Ended up needing to work tomorrow so I had to come home

From helping with my parents and getting the kids to the in-laws and I am home alone tonight. Been writing like crazy for 2 hrs then jumped in the pool came inside and here I am.

Despite all the drama in the past week this is one funny moment, a pocket of happy.

Now I promise to shower and put on clothes

This was a text message to my tribe of five after I was in radio silence for the week. Despite knowing that sharing what's going on in my life is a necessary way to get through it, I had no desire to discuss the crap that I was dealing with that week. But I couldn't stay under a rock indefinitely, and this was the text message that marked my reentry. The pivot was a pocket of happy. Yes, mine had to do with being naked and drinking, which may be very different from yours. You do you, I'll do me. And because I know there are some of you who are thinking... "She was naked AND drinking? Dear Jesus, help this woman," let me reassure you this chapter ends with a prayer. No fast track to hell for me just yet.

The week leading up to this pocket had revolved around hard spots in my sixteen-year marriage, a two-year-old that refused to sleep, a nine-year-old with confidence issues, a mother with dementia, uncertain finances, a career that was out of my control, and an overall feeling that the weight of the world was on my shoulders and I couldn't catch my breath. You know weeks like these, days like these. It may be every day. All you want to do is go back to bed but even sleep can't bring you rest. As tired as you may be from whatever demons you have been fighting, you can't let each new day be doomed because of the night before. Or the day before. Or the weeks before. Or the year before! It's easy to get caught in the downward spiral of a tough day strung together by another and another. It's hard work to snap out of it and look for the miracles in each new day, or as I like to call them: pockets of happy. But that's exactly what you need to do.

Take off your clothes and grab the shaker.

Okay, maybe that's just more of a metaphor than a reality.

One of my very best friends is a mom of five. That alone sounds unmanageable but add in the fact that her oldest has severe special needs and the others are two sets of twins and you have a level of craziness that would be impossible for most. She and her husband are amazing. And from the outside, they honestly seem perfect. She always looks gorgeous and pulled together and she's unyieldingly kind and helpful to everyone despite what she might be going through. It's an honor that she shows me the truth and lets me try to support her when, most days, she is barely keeping her head above water. She and her husband both work full-time to support their family and to pay for the special school where their daughter lives. This child is twenty years old but has the capabilities of a toddler. This wait is one this family will never see to its end. A lifetime of waiting for what will happen next and how they will manage. A rough day for her, especially when her special needs daughter is home, would leave any of us rocking back and forth in the corner, begging for mercy. Somehow, she finds pockets of happy. It's a phrase she once used when I was explaining how difficult a time I was having with my mom, and it helped me shift my perspective.

For my friend it is a life sentence of uncertainty and fear with a special needs child. For you it could be the death of a spouse, divorce, prison time, bankruptcy—any number of difficult waits that could last indefinitely. You likely know someone who has been defined by that type of loss. They never come out of the pain. Their rough days or nights turn into years or decades where the joy never returns. They *became* their wait: a permanent state of mourning. We can't judge because we haven't been there. We can see how easy it would be to disappear in grief because we have felt extreme loss. We can also recognize a desire in ourselves, no matter how bleak our outcomes look, to not become that person.

Even on your toughest days, recognize when your mood shifts to positive, even if it's just for a moment. Look for your smile. Start to laugh through the most catastrophic of situations. These are pockets of happy. They can be so small, and in the beginning they will be. You might really have to push yourself to find them. Despite all that seems wrong, or the dread you may have for the day to come, find one silver lining. It could just be the excitement of knowing this day will end and you will get to go back to sleep in eighteen hours. At least a couple times a month, all I can find to get excited about is my second cup of coffee. But you know what, that's something! I *get* to have coffee! Hot, yummy, black coffee that makes me pause and breathe and feel like all is well for a few glorious moments. Maybe it's a hug from a child or a spouse. Maybe you convince yourself to be excited about something that you wouldn't usually consider: a meeting at work, lunch, driving *away* from work, putting on your favorite shoes. Yeah, I know, I'm stretching, but you need to stretch when everything seems to be shrinking.

Every night, write down what went right. The five things you are thankful for in the day, the five times you smiled. There may be days when it seems impossible. You can't find one redeeming thing to celebrate. That's when you need to look even deeper. The sun, the trees, clean drinking water, a pen to write with. I'm not saying you don't have every right to beg for deliverance and grieve your current situation. You do, and there is time for mourning in every day if it's what you need. Sadness is really so much easier than glee. It becomes comfortable and reassuring, the one thing you can count on. You just need to start to find the opposite emotion before it becomes the *only* thing you count on.

Pockets of happy are always there. The more you practice recognizing them, the more of them you will find. One day you will discover that the situation you thought was unbearable is actually filled with opportunity and your normally rampant emotional fears when life gets stressful are actually calm and collected observations. Don't be surprised if it takes what seems like forever to get to this place. A spot where the pockets are bigger than the pants. Instead, celebrate when you are basking in sunshine and rainbows as you sit in front of a raging storm. And give yourself grace when you stop and scold yourself for smiling through a painful situation. Some of us feel programmed to worry. When it's a pretty dire circumstance and we find ourselves *not* worrying, we can feel guilty because somewhere deep inside we believe worrying helps control the situation. Remember how we feel about control? It doesn't exist and you, most assuredly, don't have it.

Don't Wait: create some pockets of happy in whatever wait you are in. Choose to see the good. When you are so overwhelmed, vocalize your blessings. Meditate on the good even if the last good thing to happen was last year. Write something down each night. At least five. Go to bed thinking of the positive. Share your pockets of happy with your friends. Send that text message, no matter how silly it seems. And because I promised there is more to me than inappropriate text messages, try this prayer on when the going gets really tough.

> *Lord, I am not equipped for this day ahead. There is no way I will thrive in the blessings you have*

bestowed on me in my current state. I'm tired and sad and cranky and everything hurts. Please give me the energy that can only come from you. Fill me up so that I may pour out. Holy spirit shine within me and help me feel refreshed and awake. Help me forgive myself for what was said and how I handled things in my exhaustion and frustration. Help me find grace in what this day will bring. It seems I'm already behind and I want to give up, but I know you can turn this all around. This life is so beautiful but right now all I can see is the negative. The chores, the struggles, my fears. Open my eyes to all that is right and good and the numerous blessings of this day ahead. In Jesus' name.

As you said that prayer, what did you feel? Be in the moment and let God show you those blessings you just asked for. The pockets of happy.

———————ॐ———————

We waited years, looking for the diagnosis that we never got for our daughter. The tests and trips and studies and therapies. The focus for so long was, "If we do this, then this will happen." "If we get to this point" and get this answer, then we can manage and accept where we are and where she is. So many years passed waiting and focusing on what was wrong with her. In that wait, we painfully missed all that was so wonderfully right. Now we're years into the waiting for the next step, because with a special needs child the wait never ends. But now, I guess in the last two decades we've learned some, we're trying to remember to be present because we will never really know what's next.

—Chelsea

4

HAVE YOU PRAYED ABOUT IT YET?

Please Lord let her be able to pee. Please Lord, please, please, please.

Yep, pee. I'm praying to sweet Jesus for pee.

I'm standing in a hospital bathroom hovering over my mother who has been tasked with urinating in a cup. I had been pushing her to drink water the entire ride to the emergency room, knowing they were going to want a sample. She accidentally took the wrong medication and after a call to poison control, I took her to the hospital. She has mild dementia and she's slowly becoming like my fourth child, but I say that with tenderness, not resentment. Okay, truth is it's hard and I wish this wasn't my reality, but I never resent her for getting sick. I can't, because she didn't do this to herself. It's just where we are. And I appreciate that I am here to help serve her like she did me her entire life. I'm glad she trusts me and wants me near. For now. I'm painfully aware that could change and will. Something else I'm waiting for.

I wave my hand under the auto sink in the emergency room bathroom to keep it on, hoping the running water will get things moving for her. She starts to giggle. I crack a smile and laugh along with her. It's a pocket of happy I will cherish forever, long after she is gone. We're kind of like silly girlfriends in this moment. I can't remember the last time my mom and I laughed together like friends. We were friends. She was my best friend. It was just us for so long before my stepdad came into the picture, and she was always my first choice. I truly wanted to share my life with her. But that relationship has long since changed.

We stay like this in the bathroom for a few seconds and I continue to pray that my seventy-one-year-old mother will pee.

It's an absurd prayer really. Never something I would see myself scribbling in the pages of my journal under prayer requests. But right now, it's my priority one prayer. I need this woman's bladder to get moving.

I have this sign on the top of my stairs that reads: "Have you prayed about it yet?" Despite knowing I should go to prayer first for everything, sometimes it's the last thing I think of. Praying for the light to turn green when you're in a hurry to get to work, or for the gas bill to be fifty dollars lower this month so you can pay for dance lessons for the second child, or for your mom to be able to pee in a cup so you can get out of a gross hospital bathroom all seem pretty ridiculous.

They're not. No prayers are.

There are no silly, selfish, or simple prayers. There are only requests of your father. And He wants them all. Every day. Every moment. Seriously, love, if He could have a constant, open line of dialogue with you all day long about everything from doing the dishes to picking up the kids, He would. He wants you to come to Him for *everything*.

There are no silly, selfish, or simple prayers.

We get so wrapped up in the big requests, the huge prayers, the life-changing ones that we think truly matter. The prayers for healing and our future. The prayers you say at night before you go to bed, the ones you share with your bible study and your family and write out in a social media post. Don't stop praying for those, girls. Keep on begging the Lord for deliverance! But don't forget about the rest of your God-given day. All the little things that cause you stress can add up to a big, fat, hard day. Those hard days string together and before you know it you are toast. You have no more to give, life seems hopeless, and you stop praying all together.

Give all the little things to God before they become big things. Pray through each one. From not being able to find your keys or your phone as you rush out the door, to being able to find a parking spot at the big box store, to (my favorite) praying the baby stays asleep for fifteen more minutes so you can take a freaking shower today. Pray about it first. First, not last. Not second, but first. Before you call your spouse for help or start retracing your steps: pray. Nothing is too silly or simple. And you know what will happen? You will start to communicate with the Lord more. You will start making that virtual phone call to our Lord time after time and pretty soon it will become an open line to Jesus. You will never hang up. And you know, darling, He never will either. You will begin to feel Him with you more through the entire day, not just during your prayer time. Your life will become one constant prayer, and what a beautiful thing that will be.

Give all the little things to God before they become big things.

I was watching an episode of a very popular reality show the other day. Feel free to judge, I judge me too, but in my defense it's a form of research as I do work with some of the women in the show from time to time. The wives were at lunch day drinking (maybe I do like this show) and playing a game of "Would you rather…." You know, you used to play it as a kid; would you rather marry Billy or Luke, or would you rather have no car or no shoes? Those kinds of silly questions. These ladies had to pick between something like being rich, famous, or powerful. I found it kind of funny because most of us would agree these women were already all three. Regardless, the answers were intriguing. One Gucci-clad, ageless woman reasoned that if you're powerful you could, theoretically, be rich too, and another proposed, if you are rich couldn't you buy fame? Ridiculous, but not the point.

Human nature is to not have to pick but to figure out how to have all three. We want the money, the power, and the fame. That's not something to apologize for. Why not have it all? In fact, your Lord wants to give it all to you. He truly does. If what you want is an overflowing bank account, a seat in the senate, or a starring role opposite George Clooney—He wants you to have it! Saying it out Loud, even if it's only to Him in prayer, can seem selfish or silly, but it's not. It's your prayer. No one can define your heart's desire but you.

For most of us, it's not as glamorous, but just as important. The spouse, that job, a child, a cure. Whatever the prayer request, He is eager to have you bring it to Him. He is your daddy and His heart swells at your joy. So, tell Him what you want. Say it out loud, write it down, do this every day and never lose hope that He can, and He will grant you your request.

Like our celebrity ladies who didn't want to pick just one, what if there was a way to have it all? There is prayer that does just that. Every dream, hope, concern all summed up in one sentence. Read this passage and look for it.

"That night God appeared to Solomon and said to him, 'Ask for whatever you want me to give you.'

Solomon answered God, 'You have shown great kindness to David my father and have made me king in his place. Now, Lord God, let your promise to my father David be confirmed, for you have made me king over a people who are as numerous as the dust of the earth. Give me wisdom and knowledge, that I may lead this people, for who is able to govern this great people of yours?'

God said to Solomon, 'Since this is your heart's desire and you have not asked for wealth, possessions or honor, nor for the death of your enemies, and since you have not asked for a long life but for wisdom and knowledge to govern my people over whom I have made you king, therefore wisdom and knowledge will be given you. And I will also give you wealth, possessions and honor, such as no king who was before you ever had and none after you will have.'" (2 Chronicles 1:7–12 NIV)

Solomon was brilliant. He basically had his genie in a bottle granting him one wish. Imagine the Lord pulling up a seat and asking you what you want. Really want. Anything. Score! But then how to decide? The ultimate game of would you rather. I wonder how long it took Solomon to decide. The bible doesn't indicate if this was immediate or if Solomon got back to the Lord a few days later. I think I'd be petrified to ask for the wrong thing. I'd be pestering God with follow-up questions like: Anything? How many prayers are we talking? Can my prayer be for more prayers? Either way, Solomon's prayer created a play book for the rest of us. Wisdom and Knowledge— "Give me wisdom and knowledge." So simple, so smart. Think about it: wisdom and knowledge really are the answer to every prayer. No matter what dilemma you are facing. Wisdom and knowledge can get you through. When life gets really tough, or the loss so great, wisdom and knowledge for how to control your emotions and fears can truly extinguish the pain. So, pray for that wisdom, and then pray specifically. What exactly is on your heart? Don't be embarrassed or ashamed. Ask for what you really need. Just as you want to make your children happy, your heavenly father wants the same for you. He wants to answer your prayers; you just have to ask.

Pray this prayer:

> *Lord, I get so caught up in the minutia of my requests. Sometimes as I'm praying, I don't even know what it is I really want. All I know is, I want*

the hurt to go away. What I think I need may not even be the answer. So please Lord, grant me wisdom and knowledge. Your wisdom and knowledge. Let me see my life as you do. Help me understand how to navigate my pain and want what you want for my life. Amen.

Back to my mom in the hospital. Maybe it was the giggling, or more likely God was cracking up at the scene to a point where He finally had to make it stop. Mom did eventually fill the cup, or at least to a point where they could test it. I handed it over to a nurse and then got my mom cleaned up and on to the next challenge. It was like geriatric summer camp; the bell sounds and we head to the next station. I kept praying. I prayed through her blood draw that she wouldn't be in pain or confused. I prayed as I held her hand and explained the invasive exam they were performing. I prayed as I looked into her scared eyes and told her I wouldn't leave. And I prayed that the next test would be quick, so we didn't have to stay there all day. I prayed that the nurse would be kind and treat my mother with respect after she had lost so much to this horrible disease and of course I prayed for the biggie, the obvious, the one I felt really mattered: that she would be okay, that this wouldn't be what took her from me. Not now. Not yet.

The truth is that all those prayers mattered. Every little prayer adds up. My heart was overwhelmed, and I was going to the rock that was bigger, stronger, better than me: my Lord. He could part the sea and cause a bush to burn; He could absolutely get my mom to pee.

She ended up being fine and we got through the emergency room process in record time. And crazy as it sounds, my heart was happy. It was a horrible experience really, and here I was warm and content. Not only because she was going to recover, but because as I prayed through all the little moments of that day, I found joy. I laughed again with my mom. I held her hand as I did so many times, but today she squeezed back. I talked to her whenever I saw her, but today she didn't just nod, but worked hard at delivering her words back to me. Because, today I was her lifeline in a scary current. Mutual uncertainty brought us closer. This should have been a horrible day full of fear and pain and worry but I went home with a smile. I found the moments of happy that are there even through the hard stuff. And I prayed about every single one.

———— ⚓ ————

Don't Wait:

- If you were in Solomon's shoes, what would you have asked of the Lord?
- Now could that very thing be quenched by wisdom and knowledge?
- List your five major prayer requests then after each one write wisdom and knowledge. See how that having could be an answer to the prayer.
- Now pray all day long. This takes some major conditioning. We aren't wired to ask for help non-stop. We're set up to rely on ourselves. But what have you got to lose? Don't stop asking for the big things but focus more on the more mundane. The weather to change so you can feel

the sun after a cold day. The light to turn green so you can get to the doctor's on time. The right words to say in that meeting tomorrow. Work on your prayer life above all else, because you, my dear, are going to need to be on your knees again before you know it.

LETTER FROM MY FATHER

My wait.

It has been a period of waiting. Sometimes you wait a moment. Sometimes you wait a day. Sometimes you wait a lifetime. I waited about nine years.

My wife was diagnosed with dementia nine years ago. She retired from her occupation as an early childhood specialist to a life of being cared for. I am her caregiver. I hired it out for a while, while I was waiting. But it was really me. Lord's plan.

In the midst of these nine years, I realized I was waiting on the Lord. Waiting for the next chapter. I had a job I enjoyed, a distraction, a saving grace. Then the waiting ended, and the Lord showed us the next chapter.

I retired and we moved to the shore, on the beach, to be close to family, to kindle new relation-ships and mourn old ones.

Missing in action, she takes pleasure in the shore birds, cackling and pecking for sand bugs in the wet sand. A shell she seems with empty spaces chambered inside. Worn out and discontinued. Once filled with wonder and strong feelings, a shell now missing in action. It is wasted time looking backward, then compared to now evokes a sucking unwelcome heart-breaking despair.

The suffering of dementia affects all who find themselves within the blast area. Husbands, wives, children, grandchildren, and parents. Direct and collateral damage is unavoidable.

You asked for stories about waiting, that's mine.

I love you babe,
Dad

GET FIT FOR THE FIGHT

Sleep. Eat. Move.

5

AWAKE, AWAKE, PUT ON YOUR STRENGTH

Cause me to hear your loving kindness in
the morning, for in you I do trust.
Psalm 143:8 (NIV)

A fresh start, a chance for miracles. Morning is where hope lives. The morning is where we unwrap, it is where we heal, it is where we learn. Progress is found in the quiet stillness of a brand-new day. We need the stillness that cannot be found any other time. Less noise. Through silence we hear so much more. Night can't compare. This life we live all day is often too much. You fall into bed depleted by family, work, and relationships. We've perhaps even forgotten all day to ask for help. Too much has been said, done, left. Simple exhaustion and gravity keep us from stretching at the setting of the sun. But growth abounds at sunrise.

Sometimes it's before the sun even breaks. Maybe that's the only time you have. It is the only time that works for me. It's so easy to sleep an extra fifteen minutes—to open my eyes and then close them again and push off my meeting with the Lord because I'm just so freaking tired! But I know if I miss that time, I'm missing the most important part of my day. So, I train myself to go to bed earlier and get up before the rest of my family and go to God. Often in darkness, always in quiet, He gets me all to Himself. Our Lord is a jealous God and He wants nothing more than your full love and attention. Morning is where He gets it.

It sounds impossible, I know. How can you fit even ten more minutes into a day that is already overbooked by twenty? But you can. He can. It's a choice. It's a practice, conditioning. Getting to sleep earlier. Investing in your health so that when you rise, first thing, your body and mind are refreshed and ready to hear your Lord. There is nothing more important than that connection. Our job is to build His army. Save His people. Love on this crazy broken world of humans. We can't do this work, we can't pour out, unless He fills us up.

We can't do this work, we can't pour out, unless He fills us up.

Morning is when the real work is done. Not the work you might get paid for, but the job of building up your soul in order to give it all back. Morning is that rare space before life gets muddled and noisy and full of all the things that take your focus from working on you, from hearing Him. And oh, how you need to hear Him.

You can hear God anywhere; no matter how frequently you ignore Him or refuse to fall on Him in your rush to hold on to whatever advantage you think you have claimed in life, He is always there. He is standing by constantly wanting to chat you up. But he isn't going to yell, and He isn't going to fight for your attention. He will wait for you to finally be still enough to hear Him. That stillness comes at dawn. Morning is where we rise and realize nothing is ours, that this day is a gift and we choose how it unwraps. He is waiting to step in when we wake up.

Let Him have your first few minutes. It's like tithing. He gets the first of our fruits in every other aspect of our lives, why is our day, our time any different? Proverbs 3:9–10 lays it out. "Honor the Lord with your wealth and with the first fruits of all your produce; then your barns will be filled with plenty, and your vats will be bursting with wine." For so many of us that "wealth" lies in our schedule. It may actually be easier to give ten percent of your pay check then to give ten percent of your time, let alone the *first* ten percent! Twenty-four hours in a day means we should really be giving God a little under two and a half hours a day. First thing in the morning. Yea, I know, crazy talk. But the payoff is "barns filled with plenty and vats bursting with wine." Decent trade off.

Don't get fired up. I'm not suggesting two and a half hours of quiet time. And in fact, I'm not even saying twenty minutes to begin with. It's like exercise. Start small. Maybe it's ten minutes, maybe it's five. Maybe it's as simple as waking up and saying a small prayer before you start the day. And if you miss a day it's okay, try again tomorrow.

Morning is where you will best hear Him and hearing Him is the best way to get through this season of your life.

So how? Decide to do it, then just do it. Ten minutes earlier one day. Pen and paper, bible and coffee, and just wait. Find a place that makes you feel swaddled and cocooned in comfort. Focus on one spot or nothing at all and be still. Declare, listen, and ask. Write it out if it helps. First, declare what He has taught us to be true. You are a child of God, you are loved, you are worthy, you are okay right now, beloved. Don't get wrapped up in the future. Declare you have all you need in the moment. Say out loud what the Lord is doing through you. He is equipping you to minister to others. He is giving you opportunity and the skills to be a light for Him. Now stop and listen. He will come. And if you don't hear Him, try again tomorrow. He is there; He just needs you to learn to recognize His voice. It's not as easy as it sounds. And depending on how loud the voices of negativity and doubt and chaos are raging in your head, it could take a while to clear them out and hear Him.

My fears are so much louder than anything else. They have to be, because they aren't God. They have nothing over me but the angry volume of their shouting. They are powerless while He is all powerful. The problem is, if I don't take the time every morning to sit with God and hear Him first, or be silent in His comfort, those fears sneak in and get louder as the day goes on. They realize they have an inroad. They got to me before I got with Him. They attempt to intercept my morning. I wake up, ears ringing with *what ifs*, and the *oh no*, but the moment I step into that room where my Lord is always waiting for me, they start to turn into *thank you* and *But God*.

It took a while for me to hear my Lord in the morning, and some days, while I know He is there, I can't hear His voice. There will be times when He is silent. It doesn't mean He isn't there. He is always there. It's only an encouragement for you to be silent as well. Instead of instructing you, He is quietly holding you. Silence and stillness are so important, even for our Lord. Even in that silence, I can feel Him, and it's a piece of heaven. It's like spending every day with your best friend, your daddy, your Abba, your beloved, the only one who will never, ever get angry and will always love you no matter what. Oh, my friend, if there is one thing you can do to survive whatever waiting room you are in right now, it is this: give Him your time and He will give you His peace.

> "You will keep in perfect peace the mind that is dependent on you, for it is trusting you." (Isaiah 26:3 NIV)

He is ready each morning the moment your eyes open for you to tip toe to Him as a child on Christmas, eager for the excitement and miracles that come with a brand-new day. He is there at dawn looking to the horizon for you. Every day. If only you choose to wake and go!

Don't Wait:

- Set your alarm for the next twenty-one days. It takes that long to make a habit, so attempt to string twenty-one mornings together to condition yourself to wake up. Get out your calendar and mark it down each day you succeed. That positive reinforcement will keep you going, as will the feeling you get from being in meditation and reflection for a few minutes at the beginning of your day.

- In that same calendar or planner, journal what comes to your mind as you pray. Write down words and phrases that you can memorize later. Write down prayers and needs. Getting them out of your head and into the hands of something bigger than you will help take the pressure off.

- Now ask. Keep those prayers pouring out. Ask for what you need, what you want, what you pray for every day. Don't get wrapped up in the idea that He already knows. He does. But He wants you to say it. He wants your heart's desires. Ask, sister, and let Him fulfill your needs.

- If sitting in silence and prayer is too much for you, because it is sometimes close to impossible for me, then read. Find a book that encourages you and gives you tools. Open your bible. Feel free to skip over Judges and Ecclesiastes in the beginning, unless you really want to challenge yourself, and feel good about your life. Be amazed by what will happen when you spend time in the word.

- Depending on your lifestyle, this can take some major conditioning. And in the beginning, you will fail more often than not. But commit and give yourself Grace to forget whatever failure happened today and try again tomorrow. That means going to bed earlier. Turn off the screens an hour before bed, watch what you're consuming at night, and allow your body and brain the rest it needs so you can get up at least ten minutes earlier each day. Before you know it, those ten minutes will be twenty, then thirty, and soon you will wish the mornings lasted all day, because they will be the one place where the pain is diminished. Your morning with God will give you the strength for another day, another wait, no matter how hard that wait may be.

———————✥———————

You're sometimes waiting to exhale. Sometimes waiting to not feel so alone. Sometimes waiting for strength to keep going on. Sometimes so tired of being the one that does it all. Sometimes I scream to the heavens why me, why is life so hard, how much longer do I have to wait? Lord When will this storm pass? I am so tired of waiting.

—Shiloh

6

SLEEP

My husband is a night owl. He stays up late watching movies, relaxing and snacking, while I'm ready to hit the pillow when the sun goes down. Sometimes I wish I was more like him. But I can't physically do it. I'm exhausted by the time the day is done. I love my bed, adore sleep. It's actually quite funny because when I'm awake I don't stop moving. I have a major fear of missing out on things. But when it comes to that big fluffy white square in the middle of my bedroom with the pretty blues and greys and the pillow that says "I love us," I am done for. Get me there and keep me there please, everything else can wait.

Danny, on the other hand, has this adversarial relationship with our bed. Work life dictates that he gets up pretty early, so between late nights and early alarms he gets very little sleep. He is often pretty grumpy for the first two hours of every day. He claims he's just not a morning person. He says it's how he's always been. He reasons he's never been a good sleeper. He relies on the TV to fall asleep, something he has done since childhood. He has excuse after excuse as to why his lack of sleep is just biological and there is nothing he can do about it. And he finishes this all off with the argument that he can manage on only four or five hours of sleep. My husband is an amazing man. He cooks, he nurtures, he loves to shop! And honestly, he is often right about most things. So, I write this with every ounce of love in my soul: *dude, you're wrong.*

He knows it. He knows his sleep deserves more attention than it gets. And he understands that his lack of sleep is impacting everything from his health to his communication, but he just can't seem to fix it. I think there is also a part of him that doesn't want to. He loves the night; he finally gets his alone time away from the chaos that is our family. I totally understand. We are a force, a whirlwind, and a guy needs a break. So, he makes a choice. And sleep suffers.

Maybe you are like my beloved husband. You are up late every night. You grow in the dark. You feel your energy increases as the day goes on and by ten o'clock, when the kids are down and the dishes done you are ready to rock and roll. Maybe, you need that alone time away from the stressors of life, and night is when that happens. Or maybe you're just hurting yourself by coming up with excuses for why you aren't getting to bed. You are tired. You're not giving anything your all. You're just getting by.

The trouble here is not honoring the biological desire of our bodies to shut down when it's dark and wake up with the light. We're talking first man stuff here. Survival skills. Our body's natural sleep cycles are based on the sun. Go to bed soon after night fall and wake up as the sun comes up. If you have pushed against sleep your entire life, start training yourself to get into a routine.

———————⚓———————

There are three pillars of wellness.

1. How we sleep.
2. What we eat.
3. How we move.

In that order. Sleep, eat, move. We're going to address all three and how they can have a positive impact on your waiting period, so get ready. But first we are going to get your head on straight about sleep because I know right now sleep is likely hard to come by. When you are worried and stressed and anxious, your sleep suffers. When you are working your butt off to keep your business running and caring for your kids and home, you let your sleep hours shrink away. When you are a new mom, working shift work, caring for someone in and out of the hospital, or nursing an adult child through addiction or heartache, you rationalize that your sleep can wait. It can't. This one component of your life will impact your waiting period more than any other. I'll say that again, because it's a biggie:

Sleep is the one component of your life that will impact your waiting period more than any other.

Somewhere in the ballpark of seven or eight good hours of sleep a night is what most of the human population needs. That doesn't mean being in bed for seven to eight hours. That means sleeping for at least that long. For me that equates to being in bed for at least nine to ten. It takes time to fall asleep, and your body is up and down during the night. Get a fitness watch that tracks your sleep and set a goal for seven to eight *asleep* hours. Lack of this much rest can lead to illness, irritability, irrationality, weight gain, extreme emotional swings, and that's just the soft stuff. Modern research seems to unanimously agree that the brain can't heal itself when it's deprived of sleep. That's why sleep deprivation is considered torture. This means the mind can't instruct the rest of the body on what it needs either. We're talking a greater susceptibility to major diseases like dementia and cancer. Big, hard, scary stuff. At that point it's not even about you anymore. You need to get your body to bed so you can be around and stay healthier longer for the people you love. I can't stress enough—the one thing you can do that will help you in every single other aspect of your life is fix your sleeping habits.

When you are under pressure and dealing with sorrow and worry and you feel like you can't come up for breath, you are putting so much added stress on your body and mind. Your brain releases dangerous chemicals when you are under stress. Long periods swimming in that junk will start to affect your health. Sleep is where you shut it down. Now I'm not saying spend all day in bed. If you're in that situation, you could be dealing with depression and you need to get help. But if you are a healthy, functioning adult, adequate sleep can be the anecdote to the weepiness and frustration and anger you feel so acutely during this season. There's a reason people say, "sleep on it," or "everything will look better in the morning." It's actually quite true. But you need to get enough sleep to feel that relief. With adequate sleep, your communication skills improve. Your reasoning and patience are increased. Your health is obviously the number one reason to get more sleep, but adequate sleep can also ease the weepiness you feel right now, that feeling of hopelessness.

The one thing you can do that will help you in every single other aspect of your life is fix your sleeping habits.

At this point there may be more than a few of you frustrated with this chapter and ready to shut this book for good and unfollow my Instagram page. I know, sister. It's not easy. None of this stuff is when you are dealing with pain and fear in your life. But I promise you can do it. You can fix this one. There is so much that you really can't do much about but give it to God, say a prayer, and wait, but this one you can. I get it: you're busy, and I empathize with the weight that is on your shoulders. I know you need another ten hours in every day, but none of the hours you do have will be as productive or as successful if you are doing them fatigued.

Our society is getting there; I can feel the swing. People are beginning to realize how important sleep is and they are taking pride in their protectiveness of their sleep. But there are still so many, and possibly you included, who view lack of sleep as a badge of honor. You may feel that the extra attention you give to your job, those long hours of never shutting down, are what give you worth. Or you see the long nights as the caretaker for a family member as a sacrifice and service you must make. Perhaps it's the kids. They don't sleep, so you don't sleep, and you unknowingly brag about living on four hours of sleep, two gallons of coffee, and a prayer. Please understand your worth is not in these tasks. You are enough just as you are. Stop trying to prove to your boss, your spouse, your friends, or yourself that you are worthy because of your sacrifice. Lack of sleep is not a badge of honor, it's a ticket to an early grave.

————————⚘————————

One cold January when our youngest child was six months old, I was working late nights, and my husband was traveling five days a week for work. I had three kids and a new (old) home (during a hard winter) to care for, plus a demanding job that had me up at all hours. I was a basket case. Sleep didn't seem available. This woman at work caught me at a particularly vulnerable moment and asked if she could come over and help. I was too tired and sad to bubble up my pride and say no, so I said yes. This beautiful near stranger arrived at my door on a Tuesday and sent me to bed. Years later, she is one of my best friends on this planet. She saved me. She gave me sleep. She let me be vulnerable and I let her serve me. Asking for help and allowing others into your mess is even harder than helping others. But what came from that is one of my favorite relationships of all time. There are people who will help you get rest. Especially in this time of need. Do not let your pride get in the way. When people offer to help, let them. And if you are isolated and there is no one to help, hire out. Get a babysitter to watch the kids at night or during the day so you can rearrange your life to sleep. That thirty, forty, fifty dollars is so much more important to your health and wellbeing than anything you can buy online.

You have a choice. Choose to get healthy so you can function at your best and make it through this struggle you're in. Choose sleep over all else. I know some of you are in the first months and years of motherhood, and this isn't an option. Take this chapter lightly, dear one. This is a very hard but worthy season of your life.

But even you know you must sleep when the baby sleeps and so the solution is similar for you, tired mama. Rearrange your life. Say no to things that aren't as important as your health (um yeah, that's everything). Take a marker to your schedule and shut it down at 6:00 p.m. When your sleep is suffering, it's a really good time to start practicing saying no. That schedule of yours could be the reason you aren't getting sleep. Before you agree to anything more, even if it's something for someone else, consider if it will make it harder for you to get to bed on time. Girl, change jobs if you have to! At least at this point, you have a life to redefine. Burning the candle at both ends, as my mom used to say, can most assuredly lead to no candle at all.

Here's the real beauty. When you get there, when that glorious, restful sleep becomes a positive part of your life again, your relationship with the Lord will start to flourish. You can wake up a few minutes early and hear your father. God wants you in the morning. He's waiting for you there. You, beloved, need so badly to hear Him right now, and morning is where it happens. Perhaps your morning is four o'clock in the afternoon because of your work schedule. That's okay too. I'm using the word morning to mean the first of your day. The time when you wake up recharged and hopefully filled with every expectation of positivity. So, get to bed. Allow yourself the sleep, because you need to heal.

Don't Wait: preparing for sleep is a great place to start.

- Plan your day in reverse. Recognize your bedtime—for me it's 8:30—and plan your day backwards. I know I can't commit to a dinner at seven because my priority is my sleep. There is obviously room for special events and rare occasions but try to guard your day-to-day routine.

- Turn off the screens two hours before bedtime. I know for most of us that seems impossible, but it's not. Maybe TV time is sacred, but at least be mindful of getting off texts and email.

- Stop with the work and the troubleshooting before bed. That's a guaranteed way to keep you awake.

- Grab a book for a few minutes before bed to calm your mind or listen to music.

- Stop eating as close to two hours before bed as you can so your body isn't working overtime on digestion while it's supposed to be healing.

- Pray over your bed. Sounds a little silly but it works. Every night after I list the five things I am grateful for on the day and say a quick prayer of gratitude, I pray over my sleep. I envision my Lord with me, and say this:

Lord, have angels over my bed, let me sleep peacefully, and dream happily, protect this place from all the negativity that can keep me awake. Help the kids sleep, my husband sleep and let me wake up refreshed. Keep those angels in this room guarding my mind and healing my body. Thank you, Lord. Amen.

7

BLACK SPOTS

My mom got sick not long after my twenty-eighth birthday. I'm guessing here because we don't actually know when the plaque in her brain started growing, or even really why it started so young, but it's around that time that I noticed something was wrong. One of the great tragedies for me in this is that before we knew it was dementia, I just thought my mom was becoming mean. I reasoned maybe this was us growing apart and her letting me go, even though I didn't want to be let go. I wanted to be held so tightly. As strong and smart and mature as I was in my late twenties—all thanks to great parenting might I add—I was still a child. I needed my mom. I'm now forty and I need my mom. I'm pretty sure I'll need her at sixty too. You never stop wanting that person who has loved you most since your first breath.

By the time I was thirty-one, and she sixty-one, we had a diagnosis of mild cognitive impairment. Disease was messing with her brilliant mind and causing her to act out of character. I sat in a windowless office with my parents, holding my two infants in my lap, while the doctor pointed to a slide of her beautiful brain and gestured to the dark spots that were causing her to change.

Doctor: Those ones right here are likely a result of stress.
Me: Stress?
Doctor: Yes, stress.

Full stop. Blurred vision. Room spins. Catch my breath. Stress? Avoidable? This didn't have to happen. My heart sank.

------------⚓------------

Mom had cancer when I was a baby. She then lived through an emotional divorce, raised me alone for a good portion of my younger years, had numerous miscarriages, adopted, then had cancer two more times. And those facts of her life are just the surface stuff that anyone could see. The parts of her family and her youth that were kept quietly in the dark were likely even more reason to feel overwhelmed. Stress was a huge part of her life. And so many of the above factors, specifically the cancer and chemo and multiple surgeries, could very well be responsible for why we were in that office watching her brain become strangled by darkness.

But the spots that could have been a result of stress are what changed *me* as a scared young woman. I am my mother's daughter. A worrier, a catastrophizer, often seeing the worst-case scenario and the glass half empty. I like to turn it around and say it is because I am also a nurturer, and a servant. I want to help others and give of myself, and when you have so many people you feel responsible for, you can't help but prepare for any problems that could lie ahead. But the truth is really more in the middle. I care, but I also worry. As I looked at my quietly weeping mother across the table and then down at my perfect, squirmy, brand-new baby girls, I decided I was not going to let this happen to me. I know I am not in control. The Lord will take me on the path He has set forth. But I can steer in response to the road.

Stress needed to stop being a part of *my* life.

That sounds all good and actually quite attainable, but for someone who had spent two decades swimming in often self-imposed stress, it wasn't easy to achieve. It still isn't. Another ten years later, I still battle that dreaded S-word daily; but I have found one proven way to get rid of the stress.

Booze and sex!

Nope. Sorry, just kidding.

Exercise.

Working out was something my mother and I did sporadically. It wasn't until college that I really started making it a big part of my life. But the reason then was to lose weight. Not a bad reason at all, but after my mom's diagnosis I considered it a fight for my future. I needed to relieve the stress, so I didn't end up like my mom. Even writing that makes me feel guilty and sad, because it's not her fault. This generation is equipped with a better picture of how important exercise is for our brains. Exercise is one of the main components to combating stress and even dementia. The ten, twenty, thirty or even just five minutes you spend getting your heart rate up can instantly diminish the stress you feel. These are facts. I mean, if it's on the internet it's true. Obvi.

According to the all-knowing, ever googled, bible of all the boo boos, WebMD: "When you **exercise**, your body **releases** chemicals called **endorphins**. These **endorphins** interact with the receptors in your brain that reduce your perception of pain. **Endorphins** also trigger a positive feeling in the body, similar to that of morphine."[2]

Exercise can also:

- Boost your self-esteem. Feeling good about yourself when you walk out the door or into that meeting can easily equate to less stress.
- Give you a positive, energized outlook on life. When life looks rosy, you have less to stress about.
- Improve sleep. You know how I feel about sleep. Sleep is the most important part of your total body wellness.
- Reduce stress. Well, there you go!

Not to mention the physical benefits. Heart, lungs, waistline, skin, bones, posture. Endless.

This is not new information. You know how important exercise is. I'm not breaking new ground here. But maybe this time you will actually listen. Or maybe not. Maybe you need to read this a few more times or maybe you need to hit the proverbial rock bottom before you decide to make a change in your health regimen or maybe, oh Lord I hope this isn't it, maybe you need to sit in a doctor's office and see the black and white truth that exercise could have played a role in saving someone you love.

---

[2] Bhandari, Smitha MD (2018). Retrieved from Exercise and Depression. Retrieved from https://www.webmd.com/depression/guide/exercise-depression#1

———————⚘———————

I sell fitness equipment and clothing for a living. I love it. I'm good at it because it's real to me. I use this stuff, I wear these clothes, I live and breathe fitness. What I don't get to talk about enough on TV is why I do it. It's not just because it's my job. It's not even because it's what keeps me at my goal weight because, spoiler, exercise doesn't keep the weight off for me—it's really all diet in my case. Being able to wear all the clothes feels good. Looking good in a bathing suit (my favorite outfit) and shorts (my second favorite) is a bonus. That's all gravy (which I never eat by the way, so it's nice to get it in this case). The reason I have become perhaps the number one fitness host on the number one multi-channel retailer in the country is my mom.

My mom.

And my kids.

I am a servant above all else, and if I can save you and your loved ones the pain I have felt slowly losing my mother over the last decade, I have done what God put me on this earth to do. Selfishly, I want to be around for my kids and grandkids and, God willing, my great grandkids. I want to be the grandma that is always there. I want to be the one who can help when my children need a break from parenting infants. I want all the little humans to know me and come to me for help when they are teenagers. I want to do yoga with them in the morning and play games midday and make them s'mores at night. I want to be the Nana, Gigi, Grandma they can count on. I want them to roll their eyes at my outfit and laugh at the way I insist on speaking Spanish to them on Tuesdays, "*Esta Martes, niña, Martes.*" I want them to text me when we are apart and secretly boast that they have the best Grandma in the world. I don't want to be lost to them at a young age. I don't want to be sick and slow and absent. I can't be absent. Absent just isn't acceptable to me. I already love them too much and I don't even know them!

That's why. My mom is why, because I miss her, and I know she would be all those things if she could, if she had known what I know now. And because I never want my kids to feel this loss that I feel. My mom is here but she's not. I miss my mom. So, I work out. It's simple really. But so complicated and so important.

My mom could have been a marathon runner and this perhaps would have still happened to her. She could have lived on an island with a wait staff and zero cares in the world and still become sick. I know we can't always control our health. I don't look at my mom and blame her for the stress she had in her life. I just know that I will do whatever I possibly can to help prevent what might very well be inevitable. Just because you feel destined for something hard doesn't mean you don't try your hardest to fight against it.

———————⚓———————

Don't Wait: find your reason why. Figure out what will keep you waking up early every morning for the rest of your life to work out. It could be as simple as your doctor told you to. Perhaps it's in order to feel better about yourself. I promise you, once you make exercise a habit, your body and mind will long for it. You will feel so much better than you do right now. Write it down in the margins of this book and hold yourself accountable. Maybe your motivator is this season you are in. In order to kick this disease or stay level-headed enough to master that next challenge, you need to be training your body. Look at the people around you who love you, those you love with all your heart. Your friends, your children, your grandchildren, your dog! Those you would do anything for because your love is that strong. They are your reason. This is another way to serve. You can't help others until you help yourself.

Now let's break down exactly how you are going to get this done in the following chapters.

———————✣———————

> *I don't think of waiting but rather surrendering. I don't give up ever, but I surrender to where I am so I can accept and go forward. Surrender doesn't mean I give up; it means I'm accepting. I am chronically ill and visually impaired, a supersize goodtime I must say, I am so grateful for what I do have. I do not see loss but the gains that come as a result of where I am, my authentic self.*
>
> *—Michelle*

8

GET FIT FOR THE FIGHT

want you to let yourself off the hook. Stop the judging and the guilt and give yourself grace. This applies to every aspect of your life. We are all human, flawed. A perfectly healthy thirty-something man literally died to cover all our sins. And now you cannot only be forgiven, but give yourself a freaking break.

If you have been working out religiously for years and have this area of your life dialed-in, then feel free to skip ahead to the next chapter, and maybe even send the rest of us your notes—if not, then this isn't going to be easy. But exercising will help you make it through this period of your life, and the next, and the next. It will give you actual relief from the mental and physical pain, it will allow you to better tackle the next challenge. It will sharpen your mind and make you physically stronger, which will make you feel more equipped to handle whatever comes your way.

It takes twenty-one days to make a habit and, in my experience, it takes a good three months to really solidify and start to *want* to do whatever thing it is that you never wanted to do before. Despite knowing about and, at one point in my life, presenting every type of fitness equipment out there, I do not believe there is a quick fix. Sure, there are things you can do that are easier than others, but nothing will replace just doing the work. You have to do the damn work.

Here's where I remind you that despite being a former fitness instructor, I am not a doctor or a trainer and you must, above all, clear everything with your doctor before you start something new. If there are health issues or limitations, please take everything I write with modifications in mind. Give me grace as well. I don't know your story. I can only share my own and pray it helps you.

———————✿———————

There are two questions I get more than any others when it comes to fitness:

1. Do you really just love to work out?
2. What are the best exercises to do?

Let's just get that first one out of the way so we can come back down here to earth. I love the results from working out, not the act itself. It's like saying you love cleaning. No, you don't. You like things *to be* clean. Cleaning toilets isn't what you want to be doing but you are addicted to the outcome. Same here. There are some workouts that I do find fun. Stand-up paddle boarding for instance is awesome. I love being out in nature, floating on top of the river, and listening to the sound of the rushing water. A dance class can be fun for me. A walk or a hike with a friend is enjoyable. But none of that is as fun as laying in the pool with a magazine and a drink with an umbrella in it. I know that if I don't work out, I don't feel good and I can't just rest and enjoy the beautiful things in life that are all around me. I get too full of anxiety to enjoy. I like the feeling of tired, sore muscles and a toned stomach. I like that I can run after my kids and pick up my nine-year-old. I like when my daughter asks if I can do a cartwheel or the splits, and I can show her on the spot and blow her little mind. I have learned to appreciate exercise as a means to many of these joys of life. But no, I'm not a super human with a brain that is wired to love exercise. And I don't think most of us are. What we need to do is figure out what we do love and then appreciate that working out can help us get and stay there.

Figure out what you love and then appreciate that working out can help you get there.

The question then becomes what's the best workout. The answer is there isn't one. There is no one-size-fits-all in fitness. The best routine is the one you will do. Whatever keeps you motivated and moving is what I would recommend. If something bores you, don't do it. If it hurts and you hate it, try something else. What's most important is that you get your sweat on, most days. For me that truly is nearly every day. I don't really take days off because exercise isn't a job, it's a part of my life.

The best exercise program is the one you will do.

I can give you recommendations of what has worked for me and countless women I have lectured, but the only way you will feel better about yourself in this area is if you do the work. Here are a few guidelines.

Find variety. Find what you like to do, then change it up when it starts to get boring. Variety is a huge part of exercise. While you may love to run today, tomorrow it's swimming or weights or a Zumba class. Don't expect the same thing to work for you for your entire life, or even the entire week. This is a long-term commitment, not a short-term solution.

Get it done early. I do recommend trying to get it done first thing. Morning is proven the best time to work out. Biologically, this is when we should exercise. It's when the farmers wake up with the sun and tend to the land. We have the most energy. It helps jump start your metabolism. We also never know what could happen the rest of that day that will derail the evening workout we have planned. Plus, for me, morning endorphins are essential. If you're in the weeds with something emotional and painful, getting in a workout first thing can give you a better outlook on your day. I often struggle with waking up feeling like the day ahead is too much for me to handle. My eyes open and I immediately go negative. It's a lifelong battle and I know that the best thing I can do, after I thank the Lord for another day, is to get my body moving. Your "morning" may be six o'clock in the evening before you start the night shift. That works too. Make it a habit to get up, pray, then move. If you haven't established that morning routine, please make this a part of it. I need at least two hours before the rest of the family and work comes into play. That means I'm up when it is still dark, and I find my spot to pray and write and then work out. Sometimes if it's a really rough morning the workout comes first, just so I can diminish all the negativity in my head.

Divide your fitness into two buckets:

1. High-Intensity Workouts
2. Daily Habits

HIGH-INTENSITY WORKOUTS

These are the appointment workouts. The cycle class, group-led activity, even yoga and Pilates classes. The ones you put on a calendar, get your butt up for and get to at a certain time of the day and week. It doesn't have to be an hour or even a half hour. In fact, there are days when I plan for a forty-five-minute workout and end up only having time for ten. My goal is to always get in twenty minutes of a good sweat every morning. Kids, last-minute work, a flooded basement, you name it; something often seems to sabotage my schedule. Even if I'm only going to get in ten minutes I don't give up. I give myself a break and do what I can, and I hit those ten minutes hard. The shorter the duration, the higher the intensity.

The shorter the duration, the higher the intensity.

I was a fitness instructor for over a decade. I taught spinning and yoga, even water aerobics. I was in a gym hours and hours each week. I loved it. I loved group exercise and the shared endorphins that made me work harder and feel better. I thrived on the people and the relationships I made with other health-oriented members. I even adored taking a shower in a bathroom I didn't have to clean. Yeah, I know, that one is a little weird, but I am also a little bit of a neat freak. But then I finally got pregnant after years of challenges and I gave up traditional gym-based exercise. I couldn't risk it. I was in great physical shape before I got pregnant and there was no reason I couldn't keep doing the same things I was doing before I started growing a human, but frankly, I was scared. I had lost too many babies. My pregnancy was too valuable, as my OBGYN put it. If I could have laid in bed with my feet up for nine months to ensure the success of this pregnancy, I would have. When my daughter, Georgia, blessedly decided to show up ten days late, and when she didn't come out at sixty pounds (which is what I of course assumed she would weigh since that's what I had gained), I knew I had to get back to class. But I really didn't want to. I couldn't break myself away from her, or her sister who was only five months old when Georgia was born. These two baby girls were my everything, and I just couldn't bring myself to leave them for an hour and half to get to the gym, work out, clean up, and get home. I thought I'd get back to it eventually. In the meantime, I ran and walked everywhere nonstop. A month became two and I headed back to work, and then a year became three, which became six, which eventually became another baby, and I started over. I never really got back to the gym. I made a decision. I wanted time with my kids more than I wanted my instructor job, that awesome cycle class, or the shower that someone else cleaned.

But I also knew that as a new mother I had to get exercise, or I would lose my freaking mind. Like literally go crazy. Two kids at the same time was hard and I was not prepared. So, my routine evolved. And it continues to evolve as my kids get older, and I have more kids, and we move, and my job changes. I continuously adapt. For me, the gym doesn't work. One day when all the kids are in school, I will get back to a gym. It helps me stay focused and the classes are by far more intense, especially when you are surrounded by others who are keeping you accountable. But for such a time as this, the gym isn't where I get in my workout. That doesn't mean it won't work for you. I know other women who must get out of the house to a gym in order to get their workout in. They need that time away and they can't do it on their own with children and chores and laundry surrounding them. (I've legitimately multitasked folding laundry while on a stationary bike. It's an art, and I'm proud.) You do what works for you. If the gym three or four times a week is what keeps you motivated, then get there. But commit. Don't let it be the last thing you do, make it the first. Schedule it out a week in advance and guard that time like gold. Remember, you are worth it! That thirty minutes will make you a better employee, spouse, mom, friend. It is a non-negotiable.

What has worked better for me to get my high-intensity sweat on with babies and a big career has been at-home activities. I have Beachbody on-demand on the playroom TV, and it gives me every workout imaginable from ten to ninety minutes long (don't be silly, I never get in an hour and a half; those ten- and twenty-minute workouts are my jam). But before I could afford to pay for the yearly subscription, I would do any free online workout I could find. Money shouldn't be an excuse, ever. Some of the communities with high longevity ratings (a big factor being exercise), are not attending online classes. They are growing and cooking their own food and they never see the inside of a gym; they do manual labor and walk everywhere.

I change up what online classes I take, from weights, to cardio to yoga to country dancing, yes country dancing—any excuse to listen to country music and keep my cowboy boots relevant. I don't get bored. I figure out what class I'm going to do before I go to bed. I set out my clothes in a location that won't wake anyone in case there is a child in my bed (there is *always* a child in my bed), and I go to sleep knowing that when I wake up, I'm working out! And you know what, I often get excited just thinking about it. I really do love my morning workouts. It's taken a long time to get there but that morning endorphin rush is now a part of me that I love. There was a time when I was working nights and my routine changed. I would work out as soon as I got off work, before I allowed exhaustion to take over. When I got called in at night on occasion, I would still get up and put on my workout clothes and go about my day in anticipation of the workout that evening. Then I would get in some high-intensity activity before I took my shower and went to work. It's all about getting into a routine and making fitness a priority. At home, cycle classes also work well; they are as close to the inside of a gym as you can get, and I can do live rides in my PJs while my baby sits next to me eating breakfast. But again, I don't always do a full workout. Twenty to thirty minutes most days, and if I only get ten, at least I did ten.

See the theme here? Just do something and do it hard. These high-intensity workouts need to be a part of your life four or five days a week. I tend to do more in the hottest and coldest part of the year because that's when I'm forced indoors, but maybe for you it will be the opposite. Perhaps your high-intensity bursts are outdoor cycling or running. In the summer I stand-up paddle board; maybe you row or horseback ride or rake. Hey, you gardeners, that is no joke. While I've never enjoyed planting and pruning and tending to plants, I love the payoff of a vegetable garden for the health benefits. The one time I took to pulling weeds and raking out the garden I nearly passed out. For the next few days that became part of my high-intensity workout. I set the timer for ten minutes and dug in (literally) as intensely as I could into my garden. Admittedly, I'm done with that activity. Something I don't like is being dirty, or bugs. My goodness, the bugs! Things I didn't know existed came out of that ground. But I did develop a huge respect for those of you that garden on a regular basis. Just find something that gets you breathing to a point of not being able to carry on a conversation. Then keep doing it for as long as you can.

DAILY HABITS

Walking is, in my opinion, and I'm not alone here, the number one exercise in the world. Our bodies love to walk! My love affair with walking started with doing a Susan G. Komen three-day walk with my girlfriends after my mom got breast cancer. My daughters were still infants when I started training. Walking was something I could do as a new mom. I tucked my babies into their huge orange double BOB Stroller (as expensive as my first car but an even better investment) and we walked, sometimes hours each day. They slept and got fresh air and I got the exercise I needed. After my first sixty-mile event, I was hooked. Not only did it help me shed the weight and clear my head, but the relationships I created while walking for six hours a day are still the strongest ones in my life. Those girls I walked with that first year are like sisters.

The second year, as I prepared to do the three-day walk again, one of my colleagues at work asked to jump in and keep me company on my daily training walks. I didn't know her very well, but I could use the companionship and I eagerly accepted her offer.

She has since become one of my best friends. Actually, more than that; she became the family I didn't have in this new city far from home. She has walked with me every week, sometimes three or four times a week, since my daughters were two. We call it our download time. We talk everything out. Of course, work conversation is a biggie, but also relationships and fears and frustrations. We celebrate our wins on those walks, and we have cried more than a million miles worth of tears it seems. Mostly me, but our tears are communal. Yes, the walking is so good for our bodies but it's even more essential to our minds. If we go too long without walking, we feel disconnected and out of sorts. We've talked and walked each other through every major event in our lives in the last near decade. Pregnancy and miscarriage, adoption, job loss, aging parents, multiple moves, cancer, even death. One year we walked countless miles through our town, me pushing a baby stroller through heat, cold, rain, snow, you name it, all to find her a house. It took sixteen months of walking, but we did it!

Not everyone has my walking team—a Rachel, or a Corie, or a Richelle. Some of you feel alone and isolated, especially in this waiting period, and walking by yourself sounds dreadful. I get that, and my prayer for you is that you set an intention to get walking and let the Lord bring you your Rachel. Instead of going for coffee or a drink with a friend, ask them if they want to go for a walk. And then spread the word. Rachel and I have had groups of five or more at times. Everyone is eager to not only sneak in some fitness but also deepen the bonds of friendship and family. Danny has walked with me over the years, and my daughters are getting to an age where they even jump in. On the days when I do walk alone, I listen to books and sermons and podcasts. They are some of my favorite times. Walking will always be my workout of choice. I know even as I age it is something I can accomplish. It's easy on your body, it's great for your lungs, and it doesn't have to be done all at one time.

———————⚘———————

This second half of your wellness routine is the most important. This is where you will see the lifelong change and biggest payoff: creating these daily habits that revolve around movement *in addition to* getting in your intense bursts of heart-healthy cardio most days. But if that is all too much for you to begin with, then just start with these daily practices. I'm a big fan of *The Blue Zones* by Dan Buettner. In it, he studies the healthiest pockets of people on earth. They have a lot in common and one of the glaring similarities is how they move.

"…the idea of a sedentary lifestyle is completely alien—every day involves challenging physical labor. This greatly reduces the risk of weight-related conditions, muscle loss and bone density loss with aging, helps with heart, lung and mental health, as well as provides time in the sun to get essential vitamin D."[3]

These people don't have personal trainers and fancy equipment; many don't even have cars. What they have is a lifestyle that revolves around moving at least every twenty minutes. These healthy communities of people walk everywhere. They garden, and farm, they cook and clean, they keep moving.

Just keep moving.

---

[3] https://www.cbhs.com.au/health-well-being-blog/blog-article/2018/03/28/what-do-the-healthiest-people-in-the-world-have-in-common

———————✧———————

Let's explore a few ways to accomplish this in our convenience-based country.

Dress the part. Make over your shoe closet and pick only ones that are comfortable enough to move in all day. I love my stilettoes and four-inch wedges, and there is a place for them at a wedding or red-carpet event. Although, these days even that's debatable for me. If they don't accept a fancy flip flop or sneaker, I'm not sure I can attend. The good news is that tennis shoes are now a fashion statement and go with everything from jogger pants to suits. Choose shoes that keep you walking, as opposed to those that make you eager to get off your feet. Same goes for your attire. You can wear sporty clothes and not look like you belong in a gym. Whether you are in a boardroom or cleaning bedrooms all day, wear items that allow you to move. Listen, this chapter gives you written permission to go shopping. Get rid of the complicated and choose what's comfortable. You can still look chic in less fussy fashion. Your mental health right now depends on you getting your bum moving. Never a better reason to shop.

Get rid of the complicated and choose what's comfortable.

Keep moving. Add a fitness tracker to your online basket when you check out, then put it on and make sure you get in your steps every day. Start small if you need. Two thousand, six thousand, eight thousand, whatever is more than you are doing now. I've been on my Fitbit for six years and my stretch goal each day is fourteen thousand steps. That's a lot! It has taken me years to get there and some days I don't make it. But I'm always pushing myself to try. Pick something that challenges you. This is the same watch you are going to use to track your sleep. There you go multitasking. Bravo.

Sneak in movement. Long walks are great for getting a child to sleep or having a conversation with a friend, but your day doesn't need to have an hour-long hole in it to get it done. Try some of these ways to get in your daily steps:

- Park further away and quickly walk to your destination. Park in the last parking spot not the first, or better yet, walk your errands. If you are lucky enough to live in an area where you can walk under a mile or two to the store, do it! I get recognized for being on TV quite a bit, but my favorite time was when I was at the store one day and someone said, "Hey aren't you that girl that walks through town all day with the big orange stroller?" Now that's what I want to be known for.

- Turn waiting into walking. Those ten minutes of walking around the parking lot before your lab tests or around your car waiting to pick the kids up from school can log you another one thousand steps and are better than sitting in your car on social media.

- To that point (this one is my favorite), only allow yourself to check social media while you are doing squats or on a stationary bike or doing some sort of physical movement. Oh yeah girl, I just floated that crazy notion. Challenge extended, now do it!

- Get up and walk around your desk or outside once an hour. We need a break every fifty minutes. Brendon

Burchard, in his book, *High Performance Habits*, recommends setting a timer for just under an hour each time you are seated working on something, and then getting up and moving for a few minutes before you get back to work. Our minds need it as much as our bodies.

- Stand at your desk instead of sit. Or get a standing treadmill or seated, under-the-desk elliptical.
- Put on workout wear first thing in the morning and don't shower until you've had a nice sweat sesh or hit your daily walking goal.

The beauty in making movement a daily habit is that you don't have to actually work out to get in a work out.

This is where exercise becomes a part of your life and not just something you are doing right now to lose weight or feel better. This wait you're in will be followed by another and then one more after that and then, oh yeah, another. Your coping mechanisms need to be never-ending as well. Exercise can be one of your biggest and best weapons against losing yourself to this pain that will surely continue to come with life. You are getting fit for this fight. Yes, mentally and spiritually for sure, but also physically.

Exercise can be one of your biggest and best weapons against losing yourself to this pain that will surely continue to come with life.

———————✢———————

Don't wait. This is a lot of information about one quite simple part of your life: movement. Just move. Every day. Move. Since I thrive on lists and organization, I encourage you to break out your daily planner and write out what activity you will be doing each day of the week ahead.

- Remember, at least four days of high-intensity workouts a week.
- Go get that fitness tracker and hit your daily movement goal.
- Buy better shoes! Make them cute, but girl, make them comfortable.
- Ditto for better clothes. Embrace athleisure, and make it work for you.
- Create an online account and track your movement and talk to your friends to keep yourself accountable.
- Invite a friend for a walk. Next time drinks or coffee come up, ask to make it a walk instead.
- Do it all. Don't wait. In fact, put this book down right now, and go for a walk.

9

BROCCOLI AND TEQUILA

I 've been hungry since we left Italy."

I say this to my darling husband as he's preparing dinner. He is the chef in the family, or as he often feels—with two extremely picky kids, one little girl who eats like a football player and a wife who is a pescatarian—the short order cook in the family.

My year-long stateside hunger is a joke, but only just kind of. Something we talk about often since our trip last fall to Tuscany. My in-laws rented a beautiful old villa on a hill in Castellina Marittima for a month. We flew over to visit, three kids in tow. The youngest, just two years old. Brave, we are always very brave in our travels. The house was straight out of a romantic comedy. Perfect cracks in the orange and yellow tile along the front door and faded colors of centuries-old paint that told stories as the sun hit them every morning. We were tucked into the side of a hill with a view for miles. There were rows of grapevines out back and two old clotheslines in the front. By day, our family of seven would travel to neighboring cities in the old Fiats we rented. At night, we would cram onto the small balcony, off the narrow hallway on the second story of our villa and watch the sun go down over the Mediterranean Sea.

And we would eat. Those evening gatherings were meant to be a little Italian happy hour before we ventured out to another darling trattoria for dinner. The spread we carefully sourced through our daily explorations was always enough food for a feast. Grapes and cheese and fresh bread and prosciutto, and wine, oh so much glorious wine. We would nibble and talk and pour and open another bottle and repeat. Finally, as the last rays of light streaked the harvest-color sky as it followed the sleeping sun into the ocean, we would pack up our drowsy village and head to dinner, and we would eat again.

It was heaven. My adoration for that vacation is saying a whole lot. I am a beach person. A sand in the toes, sun on my face kind of gal. But this holiday was as close to Jesus as one could get. (While still having to care for young kids because, yeah, if I had to decide, I may choose starving on a desert island over Italy if the critical factor was a few days with or without kids.)

When we got to Italy, I was about ten months into having completely changed the way I ate. At forty years old, I had probably done this about fifteen times in my life. In my teens I became a vegetarian, not really as a result of the animal products but to avoid the French fries I always ordered with my hamburgers at Carl's Jr. Living in France in college, I subsisted on bread, brie, wine, and cigarettes. Through my engagement to my husband, I was doing a macrobiotic diet. He would prepare me all sorts of different sea plants and I bought a rice cooker and filled my pantry with tahini and tamari. When I finally got pregnant, my body insisted on meat, and my husband finally had the red meat loving wife he always wanted. Poor guy, he had to know that wouldn't last.

I'd always, save for my France days as a student, tried to avoid carbs and sugar, but would tighten things up to lose a few pounds for a photoshoot or special event and then loosen the reins a bit. I matured from a chubby teenager, to a young adult who always battled ten extra pounds, to a fitness instructor and then, after I gained and lost sixty pounds, a mom who got to a size that looked pretty okay for TV. No one would say I had a weight problem. In fact, I don't even like the word *problem* when it comes to size. Size isn't the problem; it's how you feel about yourself that's the problem. I always struggled. My memories of weight consciousness are my earliest memories. I had to be six or seven. Horrible I know, and I sadly don't feel like I've done much better with my girls. As much as we try to shield them from body-conscious America, it's a battle none of us can really win. These days we talk about being strong and healthy, whereas in the nineties and two-thousands it was more about being thin, but the little girls see it even more today. We just have to pray we can give them a message that encourages health above all.

Size isn't the problem; it's how you feel about yourself that's the problem.

I don't think much would have changed for me had it not been for an opportunity to sell a weight loss program at work. The ability to describe products to people is a talent and responsibility I take very seriously. I can do my job infinitely better if I have actually used the product, and not just once, but experienced it in my life. My home is a legit fun house. Not as in "we're having so much fun," though I like to think we are, but as in, "I'm not sure I should go in there because there are crazy mirrors and scary clowns inside." If something I bring home provides relief, structure, ease, or happiness in my upside-down world then I know I have a winner. I truly attempt to try everything that comes across my desk. I want to be able to tell the stories that come with the product.

This weight loss program had been around for decades and I'd never been able to give it a go when I presented it before. This time it was after the holidays, I was feeling a little extra "cheer," and I decided I could commit to strictly following the plan for thirty days. This was the beginning of the most important change in my health since I made exercise a priority back in college.

Let me be perfectly clear. I didn't *need* to lose weight. I wasn't going on a diet; I was doing my job. I had a desire to shake things up and feel better about myself. The plan I followed isn't important—it was only the catalyst for the change I craved. This program happens to work great, but it may not be the answer for everyone. For me, it pushed me off my path. Forced me to try different foods, look at my portions, and it cut out a bunch of junk for thirty days. That was long enough to retrain my body and help me start craving the foods that my body was meant to eat.

We are born craving breastmilk and that's about it. Most likely as a baby you would eat a bit of anything that was introduced. It was as you got older that your tastes were developed. We absolutely train our taste buds. And even at forty, sixty, eighty years old you can retrain them.

I ditched cheese, and major amounts of carbs. I never drank soda, but that was out too, as was alcohol for the first week (I can't be a part of an alcohol fast for too long and I refuse to apologize or explain… three kids, two jobs, no cheese…just saying). That was truly the main gist. The rest was balance. This program had me eating packaged food for a while and supplementing with lots of veggies and extra protein. I had gone to black coffee years before, so I didn't miss my cream. I could still have occasional dessert because I love chocolate and couldn't be forever without it. After the first week, I learned that tequila was going to be my go-to cocktail. Low calories, probiotics, caffeine, and it can actually curb your appetite. That was it. I was in.

Before you roll your eyes and cover your mouth in a vomitous reaction to that trip to Mexico or bachelorette party where you had too many margaritas and made some regrettable mistakes, let me explain. Around the same time I was trying this diet program, I was working with an uber famous celeb. She had become a household name from a classic sitcom in the seventies. Since then she has written books, sold fitness products, and become somewhat of a health expert. She is also a genuine and hilarious human being. I adore working with her. After a show I was chatting with her, and she said one of her habits was a glass of sipping tequila in the bath with her husband at night—let's hold off on the husband and the bath part because that right there needs a book in itself, and let's focus on what they are drinking to get to a point where they want to spend the evening in the bath together. I had assumed vodka was the cleanest and healthiest alcohol, and when I mentioned that to her, she answered, "Do you want to look like a potato or a cactus?" Vodka comes from potatoes, tequila from cactus.

"Do you want to look like a potato or a cactus?"

Well played funny lady, well played. If I could look like her at her age and most importantly, be as happy as she is at this phase of her life, I'll buy what she is selling and drink what she's drinking!

There are some rules. This is not spring break. We're talking good, clean tequila. Not from the cheap section, not in a plastic bottle or what you generously pour into a margarita. Tequila can be extremely tasty poured over lots of ice and limes. It's a sipping drink, so you actually drink less than other beverages. It will also keep you going through the evening. I read an article from another famous actress who said it was what she chose for weddings and nights out because, unlike wine, it kept her awake and she drank less. And yet another super famous model-turned-actress I worked with said her drink of choice was also tequila. Maybe these Hollywood women are on to something? Now repeat after me: *sip* like a lady, no chugging here.

I feel like I just wrote a whole lot about drinking. I am in fact judging myself at this point. But again, let me explain. A huge part of eating well is keeping a clean diet, which is what this is all about. This is not about being skinny, but being healthy and eating well to keep you strong mentally and physically so you can survive whatever waiting period you are in and get to an age where you can enjoy a glass of tequila in the bath with your husband of fifty years. That means being able to eat right during times of stress, or celebration, or on a Tuesday at four when your boss just sent you an email that equated to a bitch slap and your twelve-year-old is crying about friends at school, the baby is running around naked and your husband announced your minivan needs a new transmission. Sure, we can all keep it balanced in the kitchen for a few days, but when it all falls apart is when it's *all falling apart.* That was a long explanation for *sometimes you just want to have a drink*. So, choose good tequila. Got it? Moving on....

When it all falls apart is when it's all falling apart.

Thirty days. That's what it took. Thirty days to change my entire diet and become the healthiest and happiest in my body I had ever been. I could still eat what my family ate but in much smaller portions and then load up my plate, and even a second if I wanted, with sautéed vegetables and fresh greens and grains. I started carrying around cut veggies to munch on and actually longed for them when they were missing from my bag. I made what little meal prep I did a priority. A huge plate of broccoli and spinach and mushrooms and beans or one egg every morning. More veggies at lunch and dinner. Beans all the time. They are truly a magic food. I used an app to log my meals, so I was aware of what I was eating. And I ate. All the time. Every couple of hours, at least. But I had trained myself to crave the stuff that my body needed. Certain protein bars and nuts became a staple, but I was still able to have the food I loved the most, like a fresh butter croissant, a scoop of peanut butter, or tomato basil bruschetta, because I knew how to stop.

I lost eleven pounds that first month and then another nine over the course of the next few, and they never came back. I will say it again, so it's perfectly clear. I didn't need to lose weight—I needed to manage my stress and how I felt about myself. Learning to eat better helped me survive the waiting period I was in and the welcome pay off was the scale reflected the healthiest number I had seen in my adult life. I had a goal in mind, and when I blew through that I just kept going. It wasn't as much a conscious decision to continue to lose weight as it was a commitment to continuing to eat clean and respect the aging process. Remember, food is a huge part of how we age. The weight wasn't what was weighing me down. It was the wrong foods that hindered my ability to mentally heal for so many years. Food is so powerful. For us in the United States, a lot of it is the preservatives and fake ingredients that are messing with our emotions. When I finally got that junk out of my body and filled it with life-giving real foods, my world got so much brighter.

It's been years since I tried that diet program for thirty days and learned that broccoli and tequila are the keys to my food happiness. I still battle with having a healthy image of myself, but clean foods help me manage. I do sometimes long for foods that I know don't work for me. And if I go there, it's only a taste or a snack. My body understands how to heal itself now and it reminds me of what it really wants and needs. Which takes me back to Italy. The bread, the pasta, the wine! How on earth can I delight you with descriptions of the most indulgent food on God's green earth and then tell you to forget about it and have a plate of spinach? Cruel. Yes, I know. But not really. I don't want you to miss out on some of the most inspiring moments of your life because you're wrapped up in what to eat. Had I gone to Italy with my family and skipped the pasta, said no to the bread and didn't sip on wine made from the same hills that I woke up to covered in sun-drenched dew every morning, I would not have gained the inspiration that came from being a part of life at that moment.

I had to trust myself around food. I had learned how to mind my portions. I had taught my body to stop and realize what eighty percent full felt like. I made food a friend, not a foe. I understood there would be more food tomorrow and I wasn't going to go without (that's a big one: the way you eat could have so much to do with trauma in your past). And when I got home, I got back on track. Side note here: I was logging twenty thousand steps a day in Italy. We walked everywhere nonstop. And the food is very different. It's not as processed; it's fresher, with less preservatives. So, I actually lost a couple pounds as I ate some of the best meals of my life. The point is, don't start a diet to feel better about yourself in the short term. Yes, my mind shift started with a weight-loss-based meal program, but it was just what trained me to have a better relationship with food and myself. This pain you feel and sadness you are experiencing is thriving on the food you eat. Feed it the right way so you can climb out of this dark place and move on to the next. I promise, once you realize you won't miss the foods you think you are so dependent on, your life can open up.

This pain you feel and sadness you are experiencing is thriving on the food you eat.

Don't wait: find something that works for you. Don't assume you can cold turkey change your eating habits. You need help. Follow what has worked for me, or better yet, start a proven plan. Commit to a month. Log your progress, feel that glorious feeling of success, and then keep going. Get rid of the word diet and start to eat to live instead of living to eat. You are in a fight for your life. It is emotional and tiring and overwhelming, and you need the fuel to get you through. Don't ignore what's happening in the kitchen in the name of survival. You need the strength to get to the beauty on the other side of that door that right now feels too heavy to move under all the weight.

Easy ways to start:

- Commit to thirty days. Cut one thing out and don't quit, or choose a program that appeals to you, and again, don't quit. You can do anything for thirty days.
- Use an app or book to track your meals for the first thirty days. After that, it will become easier.
- Eat mostly veggies. If you have seconds, make it only veggies. This will take some creativity in the kitchen because if you don't like greens, you need to figure out how to cook them so you will. If you need further evidence that a veggie-based diet is the answer, look at the bible. Daniel in the first chapter of his book proves this point.

"Please test your servants for ten days: Give us nothing but vegetables to eat and water to drink. Then compare our appearance with that of the young men who eat the royal food and treat your servants in accordance with what you see." So, he agreed to this and tested them for ten days. At the end of the ten days they looked healthier and better nourished than any of the young men who ate the royal food. So, the guard took away their choice food and the wine they were

to drink and gave them vegetables instead."
Daniel 1:12–16 (NIV)

- Portions! Enough said. Google portion sizes and follow the rules. It will seem insane at first, but you will learn.
- Stop eating at eighty percent full. Your body needs to catch up and send your brain the message that it's full, so take a break and stop at eighty. This is so important that it is still, to this day, something I write down in my journal every morning. I love food, but I always need to remind myself to stop.
- Drink good sipping tequila or a glass of wine if you must have a drink.
- Stop eating at least two hours before bed. Night is my weakness. I set the clock at 7:00 p.m. for a hard stop. That's about two hours before I go down. This has evolved to pushing it to six some days and an occasional partial fast. That's a big idea and there are many more articles and books you can read, including *The Blue Zones*, that can give you more information, but the CliffsNotes version is this: there is a benefit to allowing yourself sixteen hours of fasting. Eating during the day for eight, then refrain for sixteen.

————————✧————————

While in remission for ovarian cancer, I felt like I was holding my breath and waiting. Scan after scan, month after month, I never let it out. I had panic attacks and had to start anxiety meds as well.

I felt I had failed myself having been through this once before and then having it come back. Learning to let go and let God do God's thing was hard to do but also lifted a burden. I'm blessed to say that while it did return, I am once again in remission though still on maintenance chemo. My mom always said "if you worry why pray, if you pray why worry." I pray and truly try not to worry.

—Karin

SHARE YOUR STORY

Eliminating parts of your story or ignoring parts
of your story denies the gift of new life.
—J.R. Mahon

10

SHARE YOUR STORY

T he pretty woman sitting across from me is a near stranger. Our paths have crossed before, but I don't remember when. A mutual friend has asked if I would be willing to meet her for coffee. Of course. Not a question. If the loss in my life has brought nothing more, it's given me a clear understanding of my purpose. Help. Counsel. Serve. Be the safe place where others can share their stories and start to heal.

Be the safe place where others can share their stories and start to heal.

She doesn't get more than two words out before she starts to cry. A miscarriage. Her first. Years ago. Like most women who have been where she is, she gives the details very clinically. She adds qualifiers such as, "I was only ten weeks," and "My body responded well to the procedure," and then she quickly moves on to the next chapter of her story. Why do we do that? Why do we rush through our pain when it will only catch up with us when we least expect? She recounts the years of trying, the months of loss. But no matter how rehearsed, her body reacts to the black and white facts she recites with instant, vibrant emotion. Silent tears roll down her cheeks and soak her eyelashes struggling to stay open. It's been a journey with doctors and needles and drugs and emotions. She's defeated, and so physically bruised and broken. But mostly she feels alone. It's the loneliness that is threatening to take her away. We are a lonely generation.

My first reaction is to tell her how beautiful she is. Even in the midst of emotion, the mind continues to witness truth. She is lovely, a contradiction to how she feels inside. I understand because I was there too, once. What she is going through takes away all confidence. She feels betrayed by her body. She looks down at puncture wounds and bruises and feels the extra weight the drugs have caused her to gain, and she sees ugly. But she's still beautiful. Her skin, her hair, even her tears are reflecting God's radiating love. He's there. He's sitting right there with her. Holding her. And as He's comforting her, He is guiding me to show her.

I let her talk, and I don't add much. That's really what she needs. A safe place to tell her story. To let it out. Unlike with a family member or close friend, I carry no judgement or agenda. Our loved ones often want to fix things for us, and that can cause more harm. A stranger can just be there to take the burden of the words that are dying to escape. As the story continues, she lightens a bit. The tears come and go, and she asks questions and gains some confidence. I share some of my journey, some of it she's already read, and she says it was those words I wrote that got her through some of her darkest days. She realized she wasn't the only one to feel this way, to have this experience, that she wasn't actually alone.

———————✣———————

When I took to my computer and wrote all the details of my first three-year battle with becoming a mother, I didn't know if it was to help others or to save me. I knew I had to get the story out or all that pain would consume me. It would catch me. I felt so alone in my loss, even as I slept every night next to a supportive husband. Since then, my words have made their way into the homes of countless women who feel exactly like I did. Writing it down and living though some of the pain that came along with my waiting period was often excruciating, but I know now it was exactly what the Lord needed me to do. Telling the story that, to this day makes me cry, is a gift. If my past can help just one woman understand she isn't alone then I have done the right thing in pouring out. And you know what—that one has become thousands. This is the moment for which *I* was created: not for pain, not for loss, but for helping others, and creating beauty through the disaster. I'm not a woman who is defined by her difficult past, but one who has overcome and triumphed. You don't look at me and see my wounds; you see the Lord's glory.

You, dear one, are no different. This wait, the loss, the pain isn't who you are, but it could be exactly what someone needs to see. Your story is a part of you. Pause in your past without judgement and see it for how it can help in the present. Your history is a gift. You survived; you have much to tell.

Your triumphs and defeats are an important lesson to those who are on the same path as you once were. This is not about you; it's about what God can do through you. You may be afraid to speak, embarrassed to share, unsure of what to say, but He will give you the words at the time He needs. He will work through you. He has been doing that since the day you were born.

————————✥————————

There are times when our past, or even the present is too painful to speak of. I know. You don't feel like you can tell anyone. The loneliest feeling. Trapped in your own head. No way to get it out. You can't talk to your best friend, can't confide in your parents, won't cry to your pastor, because if they knew they would be ashamed. Not them; that's how you feel—shameful, embarrassed, broken—they would be disappointed…sympathetic…judgmental…who knows?

Maybe that's worse?

So, you suffer alone, no matter how hard it is to hold it together. And currently, it seems impossible. You pray that you alone can figure it out, get back to good. Begging the Lord for the strength you need to stand up even when you are on your knees. You tell yourself time will heal. God will prevail, and you will learn from this. And then the wave of despair returns, and you feel hopeless in your future. Even as you know in your heart, God will never let you down.

Never.

You recognize the Lord didn't create you to be a solitary being, yet you fight against it. Your mind is all anxiety and anger and dread and pain. You feel so desperately alone, without your friends, without your family, without your spouse to talk to.

Hollow.

You're a servant, a wife, a mom, and employee, you reason there is no space for this helplessness. So, you must do what you thought you could never do and tell someone. Confide in a friend, ask for help, spell it out slowly and hold your breath waiting for what happens next, because if you don't share your pain, it will slowly destroy you.

There's nothing more damaging to your soul than cutting it off from others.

What results is release. Exhaling. There's not only support in others but understanding. What is happening to you has happened to them. The things that seem utterly horrible and hurtful and unspeakable are in fact so common. We have all been hiding our dark spots for fear of judgement. We think our trouble is so unique, but it is human. We may not all have the same stories, but our situations are alike. We're all flawed, broken, we all struggle. More than anything we need each other.

The truth is that holding on and keeping your secrets is what's hurting you.

The truth is maybe the reason you are in this pain now is to help someone else share their story and finally come up for air.

If you have been hiding what has happened because you are ashamed, afraid of judgment, or simply because it hurts too much, I beg of you, work through your own ego. Every forced laugh or smiling social media post is a lie. In the process of burying your story, you are inadvertently hurting so many people around you. Loved ones, friends, even strangers. They see you displaying perfection when you are really drowning, just like they are. Stop for a minute and think of how you feel when others seem so pulled together. You assume they have this idyllic life that you then strive for. But it's unattainable. If you could pull back the layers of disguise, you'd likely see someone just like you, waiting through another season. Full of the same aches and angers that we all have. Oh, what comfort we find in not being alone. Not being the only one.

———————✣———————

At the end of my time with this mother in waiting, I ask if I can pray for her. Even after nearly four decades of willful Christianity, I still become uncomfortable when the Lord tells me I need to minister or pray for someone who doesn't really know Him. I'm much better looking into a camera and preaching or standing on a stage giving Jesus to a room of strangers. This one-on-one puts a spotlight on my perceived incompetence. I know it's not me, it's the Lord speaking through me but, more often than not when the moment arises, I still roll my eyes at our God and tell Him He has the wrong girl, allowing my ego to get in the way. As expected, He rolls his eyes right back and always gives the person in front of me exactly what they need.

This time I began to pray, and the words got stuck. A stumbling, incoherent mess of verbs, adjectives, and nouns strung together in no particular order. I wish I could actually write out this prayer for you because it was that bad. For two excruciating, sweat-inducing minutes I prayed a prayer so disjointed I can't even recreate the sounds. It's like throwing a bucket of paint into a fan. Impossible to make the same mess twice. I do recall having a bit of an out-of-body experience. Looking down at myself from above, holding the hand of this broken girl trying to give her comfort and wondering what the hell I was doing. I was just as broken as her. If this was her first glimpse of God, she was sure to run the other way.

That experience could have easily turned me off of praying for anyone ever again, but here I am writing a book full of prayers. Ironic. The thing is, in that moment I was real. My gibberish was likely reassuring to a woman who felt she was incapable of even forming complete sentences through her pain. Or maybe something in the small words and hiccups spoke to her more than I'll ever know. Likely she just went home and laughed about it with her husband, but hey, she laughed, and that's a win. I do know she came back to me, asking for more, seeking that safe place our Lord has given her in me.

Maybe you are that beautiful girl. Ready to pour out, but as of now, unable to tell anyone. You aren't even looking for solutions, but just for someone to listen. You have this need to get out all you are holding in. The weight is too much to carry alone. Find your person. You don't need them to give you a solution or even a shoulder to cry on—you just need to say the words that are trapped inside. You need to talk about the bad things, the hard things, the shameful things and release them. Just release them. Then walk away if you need to. Give it away. There is such relief that comes from telling your story.

Don't wait: share your story. It doesn't have to be on a grand scale. You don't need to tell strangers or write a book but find someone with whom you can just say the words. Your story is waiting to be told. To help others, but more importantly to help you. No matter how horrible it feels in your head and your heart, I promise you someone else has been there and they can help you see your way to the other side.

———————✤———————

*The maze of waiting through our infertility jour-
ney… At times it feels overwhelming, suffocating
and isolating, but somehow also it feels hopeful. It
is a constant rollercoaster of emotion and a true test
of our inner strength. I try to stay positive, but not
too positive because the letdown of another failed
cycle could be worse. Then I beat myself up for being
too negative, so I try to think positively again. It
feels as though we have spent two years on standby,
constantly waiting, feeling like we can't make plans
because what if? We are still waiting. But if this process has taught me anything, it is that my marriage
is stronger than I ever thought possible. My husband
and I, both individually and together, are tough as
nails. We will survive no matter what. Sometimes
you just need to be patient. I remember this quote
from Craig Bruce, "You usually have to wait for that
which is worth waiting for."*

—*Caitlin*

Update: A year and a half after our tearful conversation, this
lovely girl gave birth to a healthy baby boy.

11

COMPLETE

The thought would never go away. It was a low hum that vibrated through my body every day of my life. That's not to say I was constantly thinking about it, but I was never not aware that something was missing.

Someone was missing.

I truly believed that two children—nearly twins, one adopted, one a result of amazing modern medicine—was enough. There were years when I thought we wouldn't have one, let alone two. We were a family of four. A little unit. An even number. We fit on roller coaster rides and at restaurant tables. We were perfect for a buy-one-get-one. The world is an even place, and we had found our place in it. Someone for everyone, no one left out.

Except me.

I felt out. Out of sorts, out of place, and a little bit out of my mind.

My husband and I were just leveling out. The storm of adoption and infertility finally waning. We were almost done paying off all the debt we racked up in our unnatural expansion. We were finally getting back to each other. But I started getting farther away.

There are those women who just know when they are done. When asked if they are going to have any more kids, they happily exclaim, "Oh no, we're good!" You can hear the certainty and the relief.

"Two and through."

"One and done."

They are happy, content, ready to move on from diapers and nap time and prepared to enter another chapter. They are complete. But I was not. I couldn't help feeling like there was someone missing.

My first two didn't come about in the easiest manner. They arrived right around the same time. The first was adopted, and the process was so emotionally draining that I was afraid to hold her for fear my heart would be broken. The second shouldn't have survived, if all of those before (and after) her were any indicator. When she finally did decide to evacuate my body, the birth didn't go as planned and I was left disappointed and depleted. I was torn between the two for the first year, and while I loved my girls and would never wish away their stories because they are what makes them, them, I longed for a storybook procreation. One child at a time. The product of a perfect union. Planned for. Loved before they were born and cherished from their first breath.

So maybe I wanted more because I wanted a different experience. A single. Less chaos and drama. Oh, be careful what you wish for. Sometimes the opposite is exactly what you need. Or maybe I wanted more because this love that multiplied every day as I got to be a mom needed someplace else to go. I was so in love; I am still so in love with my kids. I can't believe I get to be their mother. They were cherished, prayed for, wept over. Two children can't possibly carry the burden of that amount of passion for their entire lives. They needed another to take some of the smothering their mother would pour on them for eternity. I just didn't feel like two was enough.

Enough. It's not a big word, not small really, it's just right, somewhere in the middle. Enough lives between our desires and our goals, before the hustle and the push, after the disappointments and let downs. It's where we realize all we wanted is already here. It's right now, resting in God's provision. Enough is what we see when we clear our heads of the *what ifs* and the *if onlys*. Enough isn't God making us wait or live without; it's Him helping us see what He has already done.

I have always had a really hard time saying, *I have enough*. Try it. It feels almost like you are cheating your dreams. Yet, what you want more than anything in life won't come until you are at peace with what God has already allowed you to receive. (Allow maybe isn't the right word, it makes our Father sound like a stern parent, when He is really the softest of them all.) That doesn't mean you won't still want or desire or long for more.

Waiting for more. Like I was.

In my years of waiting to become a mother there was never a moment when I stopped wanting a baby. I wanted more. More family, more snuggles, more kisses, and I had more love to give!

And as my husband and I struggled for over a decade to make ends meet and pay off adoption and various other loans, I didn't reach a point where I was happy with our debt. I wanted more for our life.

In all those big situations and all the little ones in-between, until you can say, *"I have enough,"* in what the Lord has blessed you with, you aren't ready for *more*. Because more could come with new struggles. More of what we assume is good can also mean more of the hurt.

More of what we assume is good can also mean more of the hurt.

My husband had had enough. He didn't want any more kids. To his defense, he was tired. I was too. We were exhausted. Our girls didn't sleep; they were hard babies. We wanted to give them everything the world could offer, which made them all-encompassing and expensive. We felt like we could never get ahead. But he also loved our girls and devoted his time and heart to them full-time. He didn't know if he was willing to share this good thing the four of us had going with another. We had a few frozen embryos left over from the IVF round that ultimately gave us our daughter, Georgia. When we moved back east from California, we had to decide what to do with these popsicles. Our biological three-year-old looked just like her daddy. She was crazy and confident and spoke a language only her little brown Hispanic sister could understand. She was pure joy. We couldn't wrap our heads or hearts around "disposing" of anything that could ultimately become another Georgia. So, we signed enough documents to purchase a home and paid nearly the same as a down payment on one to get our three embryos from California to Pennsylvania. We quietly went back into fertility treatments and apprehensively attempted to get pregnant again. While I wanted another baby, I was scared. I feared I was setting myself up for more of the hard. More heartache, more miscarriage, more fear. They were the big three in our fertility journey. Even though we had succeeded with Georgia, I was waiting to fail again.

Waiting to fail.

We implanted one. Twins were off the table. We could handle three but four, God bless those babies, they would have leveled us. Doctors, injections, bedrest, then waiting, and the answer was ultimately no. Our embryo was gone. Our fertile embryo transfer was not successful. We quietly mourned that baby but not in the way we had seven years earlier when each unsuccessful attempt, each miscarriage, rocked us to our core. We were in a different space. We had our girls. We knew we were blessed, honestly, we were so busy, and did I mention tired? But there was still a loss.

We waited a month and went again with the last two. Dan was still not fully on board with another baby, or with watching his wife suffer through more fertility treatments, but he couldn't dispose of or donate our last two embryos. We threw up our hands and went for it, giving God the ultimate decision. It sounded like a good idea, but not in that way. This wasn't a game; we weren't asking God to roll the dice. Our mindset at this time is not one to be emulated. The Lord gives you the tools to make decisions based on the information presented. Yes, he will establish your path, but you must trust where he is taking you by committing to the decision. When you beg God to just make the decision easy or give you a sign that you are doing the right thing, you aren't trusting He has already given you the answer. Life is not always easy, it's *rarely* easy, but the better you get at trusting the Lord and making the decision, the better you will get at making it through the hard.

The better you get at trusting the Lord and making the decision, the better you will get at making it through the hard.

"I just can't watch you on the floor again in all that pain," Danny said through bloodshot eyes one night as we were again trying to decide what to do. "It's not just about another baby, it's about what it did to you."

"But I'm willing to do it again," I begged.

"But I'm not!" He returned, tears now slowly dripping down his face.

"Babe," I moved toward him to comfort him.

"No," he said, as he backed away. "Maybe you blocked it out. You don't remember. You were in so much…" He stopped, unable to complete the words through his own memory of the nights I spent losing our babies.

Danny had survived his own waiting period. Watching me physically and emotionally suffer year after year while we tried to start a family. The pain for me, while excruciating at times, was nothing compared to the torture on my heart. But my loving, emotional, tough husband had to wait for me to live through each loss. He did not want to go back into that room, helpless and alone, and wait for the love of his life to survive.

But he did.

We did.

He loved me and our family enough to try again; he knowingly accepted that this decision could put us back in a very dark place.

We took our last two, now five-year-old embryos and implanted them on a cold, sunny January day. I felt hopeful, as I had through the other procedures. The weight wasn't as heavy. If this didn't work, I knew we would be okay.

But it did.

Two weeks later we found out we were pregnant. We were in the car with both kids on our way to an overnight skiing trip. Dan and I were floored. I'm not sure we really expected it to work. The emotions were so different this time. I was excited and scared but also extremely aware of what Dan was going through. Waiting for him to process.

Let me stop here. My story, or rather Ben's story, will unfold throughout the next pages. This part is hard to write. It is full of loss and trauma but also such redemption and joy. I encourage you to share your story, so I am going to share mine. But this book is not about our adoption and procreation journey; that book was already written. When I wrote *5 Months Apart*, it was meant to help couples going through infertility and adoption. If your waiting period right now involves expanding your family, please read that book. It will give you hope and show you how to cope. Even as that book went to print, I knew our story wasn't over. I knew I needed to tell what happened next, but I didn't personally want to go through the pain of retelling some of the most painful stories of my life. I wasn't ready, until now. Here is the change: the lessons we learned during the waits we endured can be applied to every period of your life.

Hear that.

This isn't about pregnancy, or adoption or marriage, or anything you will read in the next couple chapters. It's about the wait. How we survived the wait, and how you can too.

We are going to go through these lessons together. I'm going to be honest and bleed a little through the chapters, but the purpose is to show you that even though we waited so long for those two girls of ours, there was another wait on the way. A bigger one. A harder one. I never imagined it could get worse than what I went through having our daughters. You may feel the same. Nothing could be as hard as what is happening now. But, oh my love, it can, and it likely will. Once you make it through this, and let me assure you, you will.

Yes, you will.

I promise, you will.

There will be more. If we had not learned anything from that suffering, we perhaps wouldn't have made it as a couple through this next part of our life. There was more for us and there will be more for you.

Don't wait: despite your passionate desire to move on from this place of waiting with less, practice living in enough. Understand that as you desire more, there can be more pain. Our begged-for first child came with her own lifelong journey of pain and loss that continues to rip me apart to watch. The prayed-for third child brought with him a dynamic that would stretch my relationship with my husband and daughters and forever challenge our family. Finally paying off debt came at the expense of days and nights away from my family, and a new mountain to climb to keep all the *stuff* we didn't have when we had less.

Less sometimes really is more.

So, rest in enough. Cover yourself in content. Breathe in and out presence.

Rest.

Enough.

Satisfied.

Presence.

More will always try to creep in and disturb your peace. But be easy on yourself and give yourself grace like our Lord does. We must try to remember we already have enough. He will always be enough. You are enough.

It's not a lesson to learn, it's a skill to practice, and I'm so proud of you for trying again and again. Just by being in these pages you are growing.

12

THE LOST BOY

We saw two ultrasounds and then at the third one, there was no heartbeat. We lost our baby. My appointment was on a day I was working, and I was told I was going to miscarry two hours before I had to happily sell things on TV. My makeup artist didn't know what to do with my tear-stained face. Danny wasn't even in the room as the tech tried in vain to adjust the wand to get a reading. The appointment had been moved earlier, and my husband arrived as I was walking out of the building. But we knew before I went in. I knew. I could feel it. The fear was overwhelming, yet I still held onto hope. I don't think Danny will ever get over not being there to absorb some of it for me, some of the weight in that stark white room.

Despite not being sure about a third child, the loss was immense. I finally miscarried a week later on a family trip to Punta Cana. Dan sat next to me on the floor at two o'clock in the morning, while I rocked back and forth moaning in pain. I kneeled on all fours as he rubbed my back and told me he loved me, and we both waited for the physical pain to pass. The deeper pain was going to take more than a pain pill. We braced for the long road back to good. He was exactly where he swore he didn't want to be again: watching me suffer, and unable to stop it. His fears were realized. But he was enduring. It was ugly and messy, and we hated every minute, but we were going to make it. Sometimes anticipating the worst is more painful than the reality of it actually happening.

Sometimes anticipating the worst is more painful than the reality of it actually happening.

The big difference between me on that dark night in a foreign country and me a decade before is that I knew I would survive. When we went through miscarriage in the past, I really thought I might die. Not from the physicality but because the emotional torture of year after year of loss threatened to break me, and I feared I would self-destruct. I imagined my marriage ending, losing my job, even allowing myself to disappear. After living through these hard times and crawling out of that waiting room to another, I understood that the Lord would carry me through the door if need be, but He would not let me be lost. No matter how fierce the pain, He would be there, as my husband was that horrid hot night while I writhed in pain on the worn hotel floor.

Healing was again slow. I'd like to say we had been through this so many times that we got better at it, but we didn't. We just learned to find moments of joy through the pain and wait out the sadness. I'd also like to tell you that we accepted where we were and moved on with our family of four. But despite the brutality I just went through, my desire for another child didn't wane.

I turned back to adoption.

My husband turned away.

We fought. We cried. I begged.

I had all but given up. I was praying for the Lord to take away this desire, to close off that part of my heart and let me be content. But what I really needed to be praying for was His will. God had different plans. His plans are always better.

My husband was sitting in front of the television. His face pained. Something was wrong. He was having a hard time communicating.

"What's up, babe?" I asked hesitantly. It was six months after we lost our baby. Our relationship had been strained. Sometimes I felt like I had to tip toe around his feelings as much as he did mine.

"We give good hugs," he replied, close to tears.

"Yeah we do, we like hugs," I said. This wasn't really an odd conversation; our family is more affectionate than most.

"And there are a lot of kids who need hugs."

"I know."

He exhaled years of thought and discussion and our fertility treatments and our miscarriages and the torture of our daughter's adoption and the empty bank account and his sad wife. He let it all go in one extended pause.

"We need to adopt. Let's adopt again." He didn't look hopeful but there was a light. "I don't know, I'm so scared, but there are kids who need hugs and damn, we give good hugs." The last few words trailing off as his heart contracted and prepared to expand.

We were both crying. He had seen something on television about foster care and his emotions arm wrestled his mind into submission. Just like that. Within twenty-four hours the paperwork was signed and we were once again waiting to adopt. Neither of us thought it could be nearly as hard this time.

--------⚜--------

In order to fully love the child who became my son, I had to mourn the boy who didn't. I don't know what became of him, the boy who would have been Ben. He's six months older than my son. His skin is darker than my child's, his hair likely a beautiful mess of black curls. I never saw him, only in my dreams. And I envisioned him often. I wouldn't recognize him if he showed up at my door. But I love him, in the way I do all the babies I lost. I look forward to seeing him one day in heaven. I know he will be there.

I choose to believe he is happy and healthy and loved. I make a conscious decision to *feel* love for his mother and forgive her. But that also comes with trying to forget the events of January 2016.

Our wait for a birth mom was about four months. Not long in the world of adoption. She read our bio and chose us. She was a military vet with PTSD and no place to go. We are an extended military family, my father-in-law a retired colonel. We felt a connection right away. We flew her and her young daughter across the country and put them up in a hotel. She was kind and gracious, but we could tell she was running from something, something she wouldn't explain. We assumed that would come in time. Our foursome landed in Los Angeles on a sunny September day. A short vacation in California we told our girls. She assured us again, she couldn't have this child. We believed her. We wanted to help her. We wanted this baby. We thought this was where God wanted us. And it was, just not in the way we assumed.

Within a month we were moving her out of the hotel and rented her a place of her own. We talked on the phone and texted every other day. She put me on speaker phone at the doctor's office. Dan stood by the door to the kids' room where I sat on the floor on the phone two thousand miles away. We were so nervous. We didn't really care what we were having as long as the baby was healthy, but secretly, we both longed for another girl. We knew girls. We could handle girls.

"You're having a boy!" the doctor said.

"Are you happy?" she asked through the phone from two-thousand miles away.

"Of course! We're so happy!" I truthfully exclaimed. We were having a boy.

She was scared. I became her friend. We supported her for four months. Tens of thousands of dollars we had to borrow to give to her and the lawyers. But it wasn't a question. She needed help. This is where the Lord wanted us, and we were obedient. This had to be why we lost all the babies before.

We took a trip to attempt to find the birth father. We had to get him to sign off his rights to the child, but she didn't know how to find him. We were our own detectives. Following a train from a private investigator we hired. It was an adventure. Anything for our son. We would do anything for him, and his birth mom.

Our girls didn't know. They wanted a sibling so bad, but we had to be closer. We had to protect them, just in case she changed her mind. Those are the rules of adoption. We never really followed them in the past, but this time we had two little hearts to think of.

"When are you telling your kids?" our birth mother asked, day after day.

"Soon! We're going to surprise them after Christmas." I explained in detail the elaborate plan we had to make the reveal memorable for our family. They would never see their mother grow a belly and deliver a baby, but we could give them this joy of discovering they would be big sisters.

On New Year's Day we sat down our six-year-olds and told them that their elves had left one more gift. Danny recorded the moment, as we all snuggled tight in our tiny living room with low ceilings and small windows. I helped them read the card that shouted in big letters—*You're going to be big sisters!* The child meant to complete us was coming any day. I hit send on the video and sent the woman carrying the source of our joy, the happy moment.

"I'm so happy for you!" she quickly responded in a text message.

We talked on the phone the next day; she was due in a couple weeks, she was ready to have this baby and ready to move on with her life. We had the kids help us pack our bags for the airport and we all waited for the call that she was in labor.

But the call never came.

She disappeared.

I felt the shift when she didn't contact me after her doctor's appointment two days later.

"Something's wrong! Please go to her place, she isn't like this!" I screamed at our facilitator, as I begged them to go find her. They told me I was overreacting. But I could feel it. I had lost babies before, and I knew. My child was gone.

A few days later, she texted our facilitator.

"Tell Kerstin I'm sorry."

Just those words. No explanation. No closure to the five-month relationship we had built. No picture of the child I saw as my son, no offer to pay us back. I never heard from her again.

That was the hardest loss of my life thus far. As was the resulting wait to recover. Even though I was more prepared, having gone through this crooked road to motherhood in the past, it was the worst pain. It had to do with how unexpected this was. I had lived with fear through my pregnancies and our last adoption. The fear wasn't as present this time around. No preparation for the worst to soften the blow of it actually happening. We never in a million years thought at this point, five months in and as connected as we were to this woman and she to us, that she would change her mind. I also truly did not believe God would let this happen. But you see that isn't fair for me to say. Or you. Because I know you have said those words before.

How could God let this happen?

Why did God let this happen?

He didn't do this, dear one. He isn't this methodical puppet master pulling the strings. He is your father; He is in you and you in Him. He is sitting next to you in your pain and your triumph. Holding you, wishing the circumstances were different when they hurt and popping the champagne when they are beyond your wildest dreams. This bad thing that happened to us, this child we lost, the feelings we had as we told our children there wouldn't be a baby to put in the nursery, God didn't *do* that. He didn't sit in some cloud in the sky and decide, yes, *I will allow this family to be broken one more time.* No. He held us and braced for the worst with us and gave me the words to explain adoption and choice and pain to my children. He allowed me to weep in his lap and He stroked my hair and vowed to never leave me. He held my hand and whispered encouragement and begged me to see the beauty through my pain. Because there was beauty even if I was too depleted to accept it.

Here's the sickening truth I had to understand: choosing to parent your child is never the wrong decision. She made the right choice. She kept her baby. I pray they are thriving and happy and she is a loving, present mother, because the only reason that boy should have been ours is if she truly couldn't care for him, if we were giving him a better life. A child should be with his mother. I wasn't his mother. His mother chose to keep him and that was the best possible outcome.

It took me months to get to this point. The hurt was too deep to see the truth. I hated every color in that picture of mother and son. I hated that I was mourning the loss of a baby. I hated that we had spent every penny on a family that wasn't ours. Money we needed to care for the two children we already had. And I hated her. I did. She may have made the right decision, but she did it the wrong way. I deserved an explanation, a tearful apology, an offer to pay us back even if she couldn't and we wouldn't let her. All that anger and sadness demanded all my attention. It possessed me. I was holding on so tightly. It was like a blanket. I felt that this anger was all that was keeping me whole. But that wasn't the truth. As soon as I got rid of it, I could get some relief, but I was too afraid. My indignation was all I had.

Although that wasn't really true was it? I had so much. This situation had given me so much. A mother kept her baby. We saved her and her children with the wealth the Lord had given us.

I was her friend during one of the hardest waiting periods of *her* life. We were doing the Lord's work. He didn't let the bad thing happen, He enabled us to do His work. I just had to see it through His eyes, but I couldn't through the fire that was in mine.

This is how I now look back on that waiting room. But I have to choose to see it that way. My mind can race with thoughts of the boy who would have been Ben, homeless and unloved, the child of an addicted mother. I don't know where he is or what became of her. I just have to trust God. I have to choose to see that heartbreak in my life as a miracle. My girls felt pain, but they also gained wisdom. I felt pain, but I also learned how to recover. Each loss is a lesson. It's all great in hindsight, I know. And I will tell you those few cold winter months after we unpacked our hospital bag and told our family we had lost another baby were some of the darkest of our lives. I was mad. I was confused. I couldn't be comforted. I was so very distant from everyone. On top of all of it, I hadn't actually been eight months pregnant, so the rest of the non-adoptive world couldn't understand what I felt. It didn't make sense. To them, he wasn't my baby, but oh how he was.

Don't wait: give God your anger. It's okay to be mad, just don't let it be the whole story. He is right there with you in whatever waiting room you are in. Whether it's waiting for the bad thing to happen or waiting to get over what tragedy has already struck, He is next to you, encouraging you to pile it all on so there is room for Him to give you the blessing in return. You have to trust Him. It's scary. I know. It's not like I was able to do it right away after that January day we lost our child. It took months, and even as I write this and allow myself to return to that pain, I can easily fall into that darkness again. I'll never be over it, but I have learned to change the narrative in my head. This isn't about not feeling all the emotions; it's about letting Him hold you up when those emotions threaten to push you over.

Sweet friend, this thing did not "happen for a reason." This happened, and *you* are the reason. Your life. Your gift to give others. Your future triumphs and joys. This didn't "all work out the way it was meant to." No one is meant to cry themselves to sleep at night or wonder if they will ever be able to get out of bed given the weight of the pain that is holding them down. These clichés that come from people who don't know what else to say when they witness our suffering are not of our Lord. He doesn't want you to go through this, he didn't let this all take place. But He is in it with you and He is waiting right by your side for the moment you come up for air and realize this isn't the end.

The hardest wait of my life is going on right now. My husband and I are waiting for an adoption match. It's been almost 2 years and nothing. From the time we learned of our infertility until now is the toughest I've been through. The tears never stop, and each day isn't easier.

—Donna

13

BROKEN SPANISH

So, rumor has it when you are nine months pregnant every twinge sends a shockwave of excitement through you and your spouse as you wonder if *it's time*. Then, there is an elated feeling of excitement as the first contraction comes and you realize, it is!

I wouldn't know. That's not how my babies came into this world.

My first was early, and the shock we felt as the doctor told us we needed to do an emergency C-section on her birth mother was quickly replaced by the fear and uncertainty that came with adoption, and the fact that my husband had just boarded a plane for the east coast and wasn't going to be present for the birth. Our second had miraculously taken up residence inside of me and decided she wasn't going to get out after all. Her C-section came with tears and anger that I couldn't do anything right when it came to pro-creation. And our third, well, he was so quick I didn't have time to even process what I felt.

When you are waiting to adopt there is a different kind of anticipation. Every phone call and email could be the one that changes your life. It can truly be that quick. One minute you are driving to dinner and the next you are asked to make a decision as to whether or not you are willing to adopt another human who is at that moment fighting its way into the world. With our first adoption we declined eight times before we were introduced to the woman who was pregnant with our child. These were birth mothers who were delivering special needs children. Addicted babies. Severely premature. We weren't prepared, and we didn't feel equipped. But then the call came that sent those chills up my spine. The one that made us say yes. Six months later, our Grace was born.

With our third child, I wasn't constantly checking my email or looking at my phone. I wasn't waiting for a baby. I was still waiting to recover from the loss of the boy who would have been Ben. I didn't think our agency would ever call again, and I wasn't sure I wanted them to. I was too hurt, too broken, too flat out broke. Maybe that's why our failed adoption hurt so badly: I knew we couldn't afford to try again; we had given every last cent to the birth mother who had changed her mind.

But, when I saw the familiar number come up on the screen that June day, my heart started to beat faster, and I couldn't help but feel excitement. It was like muscle memory. Those ten digits on my screen had made me a mother years ago, and they had the power to do it again. Even if I wasn't sure it was what I wanted.

Within ten minutes, I was on a conference call speaking broken Spanish with a woman who was thirty-seven weeks pregnant and lived twenty minutes from where I had pulled over on the side of the highway. This was remarkable because our facilitator was in California and we were in Philadelphia. Our agency had never had a birth mom in Pennsylvania. Our babies were all born on the west coast. This woman was just minutes away, and she needed help.

"*Estas seguro? Es muy importante tu no quieres esta bebé.*" I fought through the insulting Spanish attempting to convey warmth and concern for her but also make sure she actually wanted to give up her baby. "*Es muy difícil. Lo siento. Mi corazon esta muy triste sin bebé.*" I had been on my way to a friend's wedding and I was now on the side of the road in a questionable suburb of Philadelphia, consulting Google translate for words like birth father and cesarean section.

I mean, totally normal scene.

I'll tell you what, that conversation was as close to speaking in tongues as I've ever been. Despite the rude butchering of the Spanish language, somehow the Lord gave me enough words to explain that we would love her child, and care for her, and we knew how hard this was for her and we wanted to help. Or more likely, He opened her heart to hear the words she needed.

There is this picture in Ben's baby book of me on this expansive lawn overlooking the Susquehanna river, my gown blowing in the wind and a cell phone to my ear. It looks like something out of a White House-based spy film. This was a grand event and I spent a good portion of the reception on the phone with our attorney. What if…? Could we…? How fast…? What's the law…? All the while feeling this hope and thrill but forcing it down with memories of past phone calls…to birth moms…about babies…who we lost.

This was a huge moment. A wedding surrounded by people whom I adored. There was love and celebration and excitement and the air was swollen with possibility for the bride and groom but also for my family. I had a choice. I could give into my fears based on my past or I could find the remarkable joy in that moment. I chose the latter. Yes, I was scared, uncertain, still raw from my loss months before. But I was also thrilled by the potential for happiness. My mind understood the plausibility of pain, but my heart chose hope.

And just like that I left the waiting room for recovery and entered the waiting room for my son.

Initially, this wasn't a long wait. Three weeks from phone call to delivery. But each day brought a different wait to muddle through. Would the birth mom like us when she met us, would she sign the papers, would we find the money to pay the finder's fee, and would I be able to control myself and not physically assault the person who thought it was okay to charge a finder's fee on a human being? (The private adoption world is seriously flawed. Tens of thousands of dollars going to people whose sole job it was to make money off of the heartache of childless couples with no care for the birth moms, the babies, or the waiting families.) We spent two days waiting to find out if our birth mother would be homeless or if we could get her a place to stay. We waited for the doctor's records then waited to have them translated, we waited to find out where she would deliver and if we could be with her. But mostly we just waited to see if this was really happening.

What I had learned over the past ten years was that I was good at giving. That was my calling. The Lord wanted me to help others. Our failed fertility attempts, miscarriage, then failed adoption kept leading me back to caring for others: these women in crisis, the children in need, other women who were also waiting as I was. So, I poured out love on this birth mom. I reasoned, if nothing else, I was going to make a positive impact on this scared young woman's life. I was going to show her Jesus. Jesus in all his glory. She would see how big and bold and beautiful my God was and how He loved her something fierce! And I was going to trust Him in the process. But I wasn't going to cancel any plans or put together a nursery. Oh no sirree, no one was getting into this heart without a fight. I was still wounded. I had to protect myself in the process.

We went about our life as it was before the call. We spent the fourth of July on Long Island, about three hours from home. It was full of fun and light and sand and boats. While still raw, I was celebrating moving out of mourning for the boy we had lost. I was once again smiling. We enjoyed each other and our children and our dog who made the trip with us. I went canoeing and we had a bonfire. Soon after, while I was happily shopping on a bustling main street, our birth mother texted me in Spanish.

Her: All good. Doctor says I'm dilated but nothing is happening. It could be many, many days. I am fine. Thank you.

Me: Get some rest. Let me know if anything happens. We're praying for you and the baby.

Her: Thank you mam. You too.

I told Danny what she said, and we continued on. We knew we were waiting for something potentially big, but we stayed grounded in what was happening at that moment. And at that moment, we were happy.

At one o'clock in the morning the next day, she called and texted within a minute of each other. She was headed to the hospital. The baby was coming. I woke my husband up and we sat confused and in shock. It wasn't the same as us going into labor and having to rush to the hospital. There wasn't the same excitement, more fear, but the same thrill of possibility. We woke the kids, loaded the dog, cleaned the house (yes, I'm a little sick, it was a friend's house I couldn't leave it dirty!) and by 2:00 a.m. we were driving from New York to Philadelphia. I texted words of encouragement and prayers every few minutes and called her nonstop. My phone calls went unanswered until finally, an English-speaking doctor answered her phone. She somewhat understood the situation but until the baby was born and the paperwork signed, that child was not mine and I had no rights. However, I was this birth mother's only support, and she wanted me to help. I begged the doctor to allow her to deliver vaginally. This was the poor woman's fourth child. She had a cesarean in the past but also delivered naturally. Here in the states it was difficult to find doctors willing to do a VBAC, and this doctor didn't have the previous records that would show it was safe for her in this situation. I was told they would be taking her to the operating room within the hour.

Thirty minutes later, at a half past three in the morning, my phone lit up with a picture of a dark pink infant boy still wet and slightly bloodied from a natural delivery. His birth mom had pushed him out as they wheeled her into the O.R.

Her text message to me minutes after the baby was born:

> *Me iban aser cesaria pero fue bien rapido* (It was going to be cesarean, but it was very fast.)

Very fast, I'd say!

It makes me smile. I have so much pride in her. I like to believe that we helped give her the strength to choose for herself. She chose to bring this baby into the world the way she wanted to, and chose to give him a life better than her own.

As we drove through the dark summer New York night, my sleepy kids continued to ask what was going on. We love to travel, and an overnight trip or a flight across country wasn't out of the ordinary; these girls have been traveling nonstop since they were three months old. Because of that, the late hour pack-up and head out didn't seem to faze them as much as most kids. Yet they could sense something was different. Dan and I looked at each other wordlessly and nodded cautiously in agreement. We had to tell them, but there was that fear creeping up once again. The uncertainty in our parenting. A desire to protect these sweet girls from any further disappointment.

"We're going to go get a baby," I said with as much enthusiasm as I could muster. Their eyes briefly lit up in the flashing lights of oncoming highway traffic.

"Really?" one asked.

"Yes baby, it's a boy, he's in Philadelphia and we're going to adopt him."

"Okay cool," the other chimed in. Mild excitement mixed with exhaustion.

"Do you want to see a picture?" I handed the phone to them in the back seat and Grace swooned over the chubby little figure on the screen.

"Aw, he's so cute."

"We'll be there in another hour or so, go back to sleep."

And they did. They were at peace. No hand wringing worry over what if. They didn't bring up the brother they lost, or the scars I assumed that loss caused. In this wait, they slept. Trusting. Accepting. Living in this moment, not fretting over the next. Images of a baby brother and, undoubtedly, the Dunkin Donuts I had promised them at the hospital, swimming in their heads.

Don't Wait: let each new experience be independent of the last. My children didn't get caught up in the disappointment of the past. They accepted what was happening at that moment without influence from prior hurts. It's not easy to trust again after loss, but you will miss the pockets of happy in the present if you keep being influenced by the past sadness. That mad dash to get up and out and to the hospital two states away to meet our son was the closest to a natural birth experience as we will ever have. It was thick with urgency and suspense, but also full of such thrilling joy. We giggled in the dark trying to get a sleepy eighty-pound snoring bulldog into the car while yelling "*como dices* 'don't push' *en espanol?*" That morning was a tapestry of precious memories, completely removed from what had happened before or the wait that was to come.

14

STORAGE ROOM

My kids' birthdays are rough for me. I love *my* birthday and the idea of birthdays in general, but the kids' days kind of kill me. We always make a big deal out of the entire month. There are family dinners and balloons and special breakfasts and adventures. We have a tradition of the birthday piñata. The kids have chosen everything from a star to a cowboy boot, even a dolphin. (Note to self: when choosing a structure that will eventually be beaten with a stick until it splits open, perhaps avoid one with eyes and a gentle smile.) Odd years we go on trips and big years we have a huge party filled with the child's imaginative wishes. Ten is not going to be pretty for the middle child. She's requested a masquerade ball with a limousine to her favorite Mexican restaurant, a photo booth, and a bartender.

She's nine.

How have I failed her already? A bar, really? Despite my assurance of only virgin piña coladas, I'm sure all the parents will be thrilled to see that one on the invite.

We do a really good job of making these events a celebration. Every year is a gift. But when it comes to celebrating the day my three favorite small humans came into this world, I have a really hard time. Part of it is they are getting older and I miss my babies, but the tears that unavoidably fall at some point during the day, usually come from the memories of the trauma of the actual day of their birth, and for my two adopted children, tears for the women I left behind.

When we got to the hospital in Philadelphia, Ben was less than two hours old. Our baby was in the nursery swaddled in a blue and pink blanket in an old, clear plastic bassinet, crying soundlessly. There wasn't this moment of realization or connection like there was when my first child was born.

With Grace, I had been so intimately connected to her development for six months that when she was finally in my arms, I felt like I had known her forever. Ben was still a stranger. I hadn't had the time to prepare. I hadn't let myself imagine him. I still didn't believe he was ours. And technically he wasn't.

We were all given black and white visitor stickers and sent to a faded old waiting room. After our birth mother gave permission, Ben was wheeled in by his nurse who allowed us to hold him. Georgia was overflowing with jubilation. She held the little bundle and giggled, and her eyes shone like the sun as she looked at her baby brother. Grace was standoffish and concerned. She bit her lower lip, a gesture that always made me think of her own birth mother. She wouldn't hold Ben until I put her in my lap and wrapped my arms safely around them both. It's hard to say what was going through the mind of my firstborn. Was she picking up on the uncertainty *I* felt over whether or not this child would ultimately be ours? Was she guarding herself as I was from falling in love for fear he would be taken away? Or was she struggling with this adoption day, wondering how it compared to hers seven years earlier? Maybe it was just a natural reaction to watching a helpless human come into your world. Whatever it was, it quickly faded, and within minutes my sweet oldest daughter tumbled head over heels in love with the baby that sealed our family. Her passion for him was and continues to be the strongest. He didn't just complete our family of five, he somehow saved her. Those feelings of displacement and not fitting in to a group of people with the same blood running through their pale skin, were erased when a nearly eight pound adopted brown boy entered her world.

The girls eventually went home with their cousin and we spent the day volleying between social workers and lawyers and translators. Danny held tightly to his son, only putting him down for tests and examinations. We had been through this before and we knew the importance of bonding with the baby immediately. This meant only we should be holding him, and he needed to be in our arms as much as possible. Some of the nurses and staff were sympathetic to the adoption process and to us as adopted parents, but others continued to try to reunite Ben with his birth mother. Thankfully, she was committed to her recovery, which didn't include prolonged time with a child she would not parent. Because she had no one here to help her, I was her support. I knew I was a constant reminder of what she was losing, and in a perfect world she would have a facilitator there along with her own family to hold her hand as she signed the papers and cradle her heart as it broke. But it was me who she had instead.

This is where I knew I needed to serve her: show her God's love by being present even though I was petrified of this situation. We had a forty-eight-hour wait before she could sign the papers to start the adoption. The minutes rolled by slowly. She would text me when she needed more pain medication. She would let me know when the doctors and nurses came in so that I could translate for her. The recovery room she was placed in was less than two hundred feet from where we were with her baby and we spent the day going back and forth caring for both mother and child. Twice she asked me to bring Ben into her room and I stayed, at her request, in an old chair in the corner as she stroked his body with her hand, unwrapping him like a gift and memorizing every shade of his fresh skin. When he fussed, she would ask me to comfort him. If he needed a change, she would insist I do the diapering. She couldn't play the role of mother. She repeated that we were his parents, not her. She put our name on his crib, our name on the birth certificate, she allowed us to give him our last name. She was getting the closure she needed, and I welcomed the involvement. As long as she was communicating with us, I felt a false sense of security that she wasn't changing her mind.

Because she still could.

She could always take him away. These forty-eight hours were just the beginning of one of the most torturous waits of our lives.

The day became night and the hospital prepared for rest.

"We really can't give you a room," the nurse attempted to gently explain. "The baby can stay in with the mother…"

"Birth mother," I kindly interrupted.

"…well with her," she continued.

"I'm so sorry," I stopped her again. "But that's honestly not what she wants. She doesn't want to bond."

"Well we can keep him in the nursery, that's not a problem, and then you can come back in the morning and we can bring him back to you in the waiting room until the social worker gets here."

We were attempting to treat everyone in this hospital with as much grace as we could muster, but it was so hard to explain years' worth of learning about infant adoptions in minutes to nurses who had no experience with a situation like ours.

"We really can't leave our baby," I begged. "It's important for him to bond with us, we need to be holding him nonstop right now," I added.

"Can we just stay overnight in the waiting room?" Danny chimed in, snuggling the sleeping infant, already falling effortlessly back into the role of father to a newborn. With our firstborn, we had months to prepare the hospital staff and rally for our adoptive parents' rights. We had a room where we lived with our baby girl for the two days she was in the hospital until she was discharged. We had nurses who catered to us as much as our baby and helped us become successful first-time parents. But with Ben, we didn't even know where he would be delivered. We were at the mercy of the social workers and nurses in whatever hospital we landed. And, despite how common adoption is now, so many people are still skeptical of the situation. Rightfully so, as everyone should have the birth parents' best interests in mind. But just as important are the needs of the baby, and that baby needed to be in our arms without pause in order to make up for the loss he was undoubtedly feeling.

The nurse looked at us with sympathy. "Let me see what I can do. There is a storage room off the nursery we use for overflow, maybe we can put you there."

"Oh my, that would be so amazing. We can't thank you enough," I exclaimed, near tears. Never so thrilled in my life about the prospect of a night in a storage closet.

"Hold on, I need to see if it's even a possibility." She left us and we waited. Again. Little waits strung together during one big wait. And this time, ironically, in a literal waiting room. A half hour later, we were in a large storage room, our son sleeping peacefully in his plastic bassinet.

I looked around at the piles of linens and medical equipment, I put down my bag, and sat on the white linoleum. "No room at the inn, I guess, right?"

"Are you comparing us to Mary, Joseph, and Jesus?" my husband said to me in mock shock.

"I mean, no, but come on, a barn might be nicer."

"You're seriously going to hell." He laughed.

I laughed too, but then I started to cry.

My emotions are always so close together. Joy and sorrow nearly one and the same.

"Babe...?" His eyes got wide, trying to figure out what was happening in front of him. Seconds before, we were laughing and now I was falling apart. We had been up for nearly twenty-four hours and the mental and emotional toll of the day was beginning to show. "Lie down, sleep some," he said motioning to the floor.

There wasn't even a pillow or a cot. Just the cold, stark floor and my backpack for a pillow.

"No, it's okay, it's just…" The tears fell quickly. "…I'm not feeling this yet," I said motioning to the air, the room, the baby.

He had picked up our sleeping son and was slowly rocking him. That motion that becomes so familiar as the parent of a newborn that you find yourself swaying even when the baby is no longer in your arms. "What do you mean? He's here, we're here, this is good?" He stated this as a question. Knowing the answer but urging me to figure it out myself.

"We're taking her baby." I paused on that thought, then quickly qualified. "I just don't know, she is sad and in pain, and we're here with her baby and we're supposed to be happy." I cried now, so caught in my head between easing the suffering of this woman down the hall and feeling my own elation at becoming a mother again.

"You're just tired babe," Dan reasoned. "You need to get some rest." He had his own demons to battle as he watched me unravel. This is the baby I wanted, I begged for, a child and a situation he wasn't originally prepared for. His heart had been broken. Now, he watched his wife ripped open in her own pain in the last two years since he agreed this was what we needed to do. Here I was getting exactly what I wanted, what *we* wanted, and I still couldn't find happy.

"Yea, sorry, sorry, I just feel so sick. You're right, I'm tired, and this is different, with her…" I explained, nodding to the hallway where, feet away, our birth mother was recovering. It was different. I was caring for the birth mother and the baby. This wasn't how it was supposed to be. Too many competing emotions. My existence brought her pain, even as her pain brought me joy.

"I love you, I'm sorry." I strung the words together quickly trying to will the moment away and force myself to fall in love with this stranger who already seemed to have my husband's heart. I curled up in the fetal position on the hard hospital floor and fell asleep to the sound of a love song Dan sang sweetly to our sleeping son.

Don't Wait: let go of expectations. Sometimes the thing you thought would fix you, heal you, complete you, will bring more questions than answers. You are putting too much power into the hands of the future. Be, rather than wait. Just be. No expectations. Don't expect your life to be miraculously transformed when the door of that waiting room opens. More often than not, that door just leads to another room full of waiting.

I went through a divorce six years ago. I have been alone ever since. I know I have to learn self-love before I even consider another relationship. All my children are grown, and I have three precious grandchildren. But they are all far away as my son-in-law is in the army. Feeling lonely is the worst. I am waiting and preparing myself physically, emotionally and spiritually to be in a good place for when the time comes that the Lord brings someone into my life.

—Carolyn

15

NINE MONTHS OF WAITING

There is a promise of light in the room but it's still not there. Mainly darkness, a milky grey weight of the morning. My eyes aren't open, but my mind is wide awake. I want to go back to sleep. I deserve more sleep. My swirling mind resists. The fear is stirring me out of blissful slumber. It's worse than a sleepless child, louder than a neighbor's early lawn mower, more insistent than a scheduled alarm. Anxiety over that which I can't control, forcing me to attention.

There is a sleeping baby in a bassinet beside me. Bolts of light flood my brain as the reality of the past few days comes rushing back. Not just what has happened—the beauty and astonishment of my son—but the reality of what we are now waiting for. The fear grips me again. Threatens to take my breath. As quietly as possible, I get out of bed and prepare for the day. Today. A big day. My baby is three days old. I am headed back to work. His birth mother will be signing the papers that will almost make him ours. Almost. But really, she is just starting the clock. Thirty days we are granted to parent her child while she decides if she can live without him. Thirty days she has to change her mind. Every second I spend with him I fall deeper in love, as I pray, mercifully, she falls out.

This morning, the anxiety that has always threatened the start of my days pleads with me that it deserves center attention. *Your child could be gone at any moment.* It whispers with its heady breath in my buzzing ears. *Get ready for another torturous loss.* How do I wait gracefully through this one?

Work.

I have to go back to work. It sounds crazy; it feels crazy. I am way too gooey from new motherhood and emotion to be trusted to talk on national television for hours at a time, but if these waits have taught me one thing, it's that I can be a tremendous actress. I can fake just about anything and do it damn well. There is also a relief in focusing on something other than the passage of time. While I present cameras and cleaning supplies, my newborn son will be bonding with his daddy and sisters as we all wait to hear from our lawyers. The paperwork is signed, the clock beginning to tick. The text comes in while I'm on the air. My smart watch lights up with my lawyers' number. I glance down and then back to my on-air guest as she addresses the talk to text function on the cell phone we are demonstrating. I keep my emotions level. No one knows what's going on in my bursting heart, and that's exactly how it needs to be.

Because of my position, and the millions of viewers who see me on TV on a daily basis, I can't just disappear without explanation. There isn't maternity leave for an adoptive mother, not that we could afford time off anyway. Those lawyers—at that very moment sitting in an office with our birth mother working on the paperwork, while I am on national television working on selling goods to America—are getting our very last cent. We decided not to announce our new addition to the world until the thirty-day waiting period was over. Which means I will be working through the first month of our child's life. I am able to take a few days off and scale back during the week but still be present enough that not many will question my absence. Only three people at work know what has happened: my boss, her boss, and my social partner who not only organizes my social media but also my life. Just the essentials. I want to tell everyone I see but I must keep it in, until he is ours. But oh, how he already is.

Each morning I wake up racked with fear over what the day could bring. Will she call? Will she text? Will we lose him? But simultaneously I am so full of such joy over the baby boy I hold in my arms. I head to work and leave all my emotions at the door. Compartmentalizing. I suck at it. But I have no other choice.

That month of waiting seemed like an eternity. I wanted it over, while concurrently wishing this time with my newborn would slow down. Twice, our birth mother messaged me asking after the child and looking for a picture. I was comforted by her communication. As long as she was in contact, I could continue to sway her decision. Silly me. There is no control. There never was. There never will be.

There is no control. There never was. There never will be.

Our thirty days ended and we celebrated, but with that wait behind us, another presented. Ben's birth father needed to be found in order to finalize the adoption. This man was somewhat of a mystery. He was presumably in a different country, we only had a first name, and we had no way of contacting him. The birth mother gave us all the details she had but they were lacking. So now we had to wait to see if he came looking for his child. We were forced to endure six months before we could claim abandonment and get his rights dissolved.

Six months we waited to see if we would lose our child.

Six months.

So many *what ifs* played out in our heads. We were told he knew about the baby but didn't want to be involved. Which could be good in that he didn't want this baby, or it could be bad in that he could still change his mind. As with all adoption issues, it came down to money. We had to take out advertisements looking for him. We were even told we would need to pay the country where we assumed he was fifteen thousand dollars to find him.

"So, what happens if we can't?" I cried to our lawyer days before Christmas. "We don't have fifteen grand to give them! Will we just have to ship the baby to them, or will the state take him back? This is crazy! He's a U.S. citizen, he was born here, this isn't fair!"

Girl, feel my volume. I was so freaking loud. My fear was overwhelming. I was immediately in the worst-case scenario. Convinced the house was burning.

"I don't know, but we will figure it out," my kind, patient lawyer explained.

(Funny fact: I took the LSAT. I got into law school after undergrad. I wanted to be a lawyer, but life took a different turn when I fell into TV. Now I see God's hand in this pivot. There is no way I could be a lawyer! They are all so calm and composed and there are no tears involved. Thank the Lord for unanswered prayers on that one.)

"I know this isn't ideal but I'm working on it," my level-headed lawyer continued.

Not nearly at *my* speed. I long for information immediately. I don't wait well. I want to see the end game before the teams are even picked. Patience isn't a trait I possess. And waiting on others is often the toughest wait of all.

"It's just so hard for everyone to bond with him and fully accept him when he isn't yet really ours." I whispered, not wanting to voice this pain.

It was the truth. I felt some in our extended family were slow to get attached for fear he could be gone. He was nearly six months old and he was cemented into our hearts. Could there really be an ending here where he was taken away?

By January we were given a court date to petition for dissolution of the rights of this unknown man. Blessedly we were granted our request, but then another thirty-day wait began in which he could change his mind. Mind you "he" didn't even know this was happening.

We were again just waiting in the *what if*.

By the end of March our final court date arrived. We gathered a tribe of people who knew and loved Ben and literally paraded our kids and their friends and their parents the two blocks from the school to the court house in the middle of the day. We were so full of excitement and expectation. We packed the court room with humans of all ages and colors and we listened as the judge and the lawyers discussed the events of the last nine and a half months.

Again, we waited.

Thirty minutes later, with more than a few nails bitten and not a dry eye in the room, a wand was waved (no really, the judge had a fairy godmother wand, you can't make this stuff up) and we became Ben Diego's mom and dad.

The long wait was over.

And the crowd went wild.

Don't Wait: the sooner you understand that with the end of one wait will come another, the quicker you will get to your next chapter. Remove yourself from the emotionality of the circumstances. (Easy for me to say, as I look back on some emotional highs and lows from this season that should have earned me a royal title.) When the news comes, the phone rings, the letter arrives, lay witness to the emotions but don't let them own you. Each morning that you wake up gripped with worry, accept those feelings, but choose to walk in the other direction. It doesn't mean you don't keep doing the work, moving the needle, finding the solution, but it means you break up with the emotional aspect of your struggle. It wasn't just a thirty day wait, it was another six months, then another thirty, then another month and you know what, once that wand was waved, we found ourselves waiting again. Maybe it wasn't as hard or as time consuming, but it was another wait just the same. If you let yourself be enslaved to the emotions that come with your anxiety every morning (as it is for me) or every day, then you won't find the pockets of happy that are unfolding in your midst. Those were the first nine months of my child's life. His first smile, his first Christmas, his first snowfall. No venomous voice of anxiety was going to keep me from being present in those moments, no matter how scared I was in my wait.

Get in that waiting room and make it your home, accept it, pack away the emotional baggage you brought with you and find the people or things in there that will keep you smiling. And when it's time to move on, take them with you. You're going to need them again real soon.

I'm currently waiting for what happens after maternity leave. Waiting for the right time to go back into the workforce. Waiting to understand if that's even what I want to do. Do I just focus on raising my kids now and focus on my career later? Do I wait for the right opportunity to come along because now I have this child who means so much more to me? Or will waiting mean there will be no work to go back to once my child is grown.

—Therese

16

LETTER TO OUR BIRTH MOTHERS

There's a woman out there somewhere who I miss.

Two actually.

They gave birth to the children I now call my own. Each woman is different and unique, like their babies. Both situations are beautiful, yet heartbreaking just the same.

One gave birth to this beautiful girl.

One delivered this incredible boy.

It was the best day of my life and one of the hardest at the same time. When I took my baby daughter in my arms, I said goodbye to the woman who had become my friend and the center of my life for five months. I said goodbye to the girl who had come to depend on me to help save her.

It was easier for her that way. So, I walked. We went through one of the most intimate and traumatic events of our lives together and I mourned her, still mourn her, even as I finally became whole as a mother at last.

I look at Grace and see her birth mom in the way my daughter sighs or cries and I'll be overcome with longing to see that woman again, to hold her, to hug her and clasp hands and look in her eyes and giggle like girlfriends. To tell her it's good. It's all so, so good. We did it.

She did it.

What she wanted for her child, the dream, the wish, it all came true and so much more. We are overwhelmingly blessed, and her child is thriving. I don't pretend to understand what is going through the mind and heart of either of our birth mothers, years later, but I pray they can somehow feel the love I still have for them, and that their children have, even if they haven't quite figured out all their feelings just yet.

Without these women out there somewhere there would be no Grace. Ben would not exist. And there would be no me because I wouldn't have survived. At least not as the woman I am today. There would be no Georgia or Dan or any of the beauty that makes us this amazing family.

I miss her.

Oh, how I miss you....

> *I want you to know she's beautiful like you and so smart and loving and talented and overly sensitive (like me) and there are parts of her that are hard, so hard, I think we both knew that at one point in her life there would be some darkness to illuminate in her, but she's worth every second.*
>
> *I'll keep chasing her light, I promise.*
>
> *He's sweet and smart and full of this fire for life. He loves his sisters with a passion that's beyond blood. He's stubborn, and loud, and smart beyond*

his years. He is the boy we both dreamed of when you told me you couldn't keep him. He's so much more than I ever knew I needed.

Especially on her birthday, I want so badly to talk to you. It's not fair. It's selfish of me.

But there is no other woman on earth who loves this child as much as I do, and I yearn to share that with you. To give you one more hug and tell you again, what a beautiful human you created. It's a miracle. You know that. You could have decided differently. But you didn't. You chose to grow every beautiful inch of her, selflessly, and then give her to me. And you, you chose to protect him, give him a better future. Those decisions saved their lives and changed my life. Saved me. Truly saved me.

We did it, mamas. We survived what we thought we might not. The pain of the wait. The fear of the outcome. The family and friends who didn't sit by your side. The lonely nights of doubt. The scary reality of a birthday. The months of lawyers and court dates and finally, the hardest part of all. The end. The wait was over and so were we. An added loss we didn't expect.

We did it. You did it. She is the best thing you ever did. He is the best decision you ever made. I am so proud of you, and I will always, always think of you and miss you.

———— ✣ ————

Don't Wait: it's okay to grieve. There is healing in the tears. You get to mourn. Please girl, mourn. Never apologize for your grief. Having God in you means you are still perfect despite being filled with sadness. If revisiting the past hurts helps, then do it! Grieve. Cry it out. Scream in pain. No one gets to tell you how to recover. Look back with pain at what hurt you but also look back at what has brought you here and made you stronger.

FIND YOUR SUPPORT

We only finally heal when we give
of ourselves to others.

17

WE NEED GIRLS

We need people. That's different than being needy. I mean, yes, we're probably a little of that too. Maybe some more than others. (Insert finger pointing emoji here.) But this isn't neediness—this is needing people. Not just any people, the right people. Real people. People who get real with us. Loving, accepting, safe people who feel free to judge, because we need that judgement sometimes. Judgement from those who care shouldn't feel like being judged. We need people who aren't afraid to tell the truth but, (and here is the heart of it) people who will love us regardless. True love for all our parts, even the broken ones. Those who will see the payoff in investing time in the life of another, even if it means getting messy and sharing the covered heart and soul parts that have yet to see the light of day.

That's not just anyone. That's a special kind of person.

My husband is my best friend and I wouldn't trade him for the world, but this is a job for a woman, a sister, a girlfriend. I've had some guy friends in my life who fit the bill, but they are rare and often fleeting. But a true girlfriend who loves unconditionally, gives selflessly, and never leaves no matter how hard it gets—that's what we need. And really, more than one.

One like us, because we are awesome.

One who isn't anything at all like us, because we can be too much sometimes.

One that is going in our same direction, and lastly one who has been where we have been. That last one may be the most important, because she is who needs us the most. We need to give in order to receive. We only really heal when we give of ourselves to others.

We need a tribe. A posse. A haven.

But so many of us don't have that. And we feel the loss as we wait.

When did making women friends become so hard? We are all so busy and have a million kids and can barely keep our heads above water at times, but why does that equate to distance from the people who can keep us afloat? We grew up with girlfriends. We laughed and cried and shared and stretched together during some of the most difficult years of adolescence and early adulthood. We were vulnerable and awkward and struggled our way through our lives, together. Those teenage years should have been a time when friendships easily dissipated as our very beings changed so rapidly, but somehow, we stuck together. I look back at pictures of those girls I knew and long for closeness and adventure like that once again. It wasn't always easy, and girls can be mean, but in so many ways it was easier than it is now.

Decades later, so much gets in the way of closeness. Pride. Loss. Fear. Shame. Every experience that takes our breath away and breaks a hole in our hearts also lands another brick in a wall that becomes harder and harder to see around. We assume we're alone on this island where life isn't ending up the way we planned when we were younger. But we're not. We assume everyone around us doesn't want to hear about what keeps us up at night or causes us to cry alone in the bathroom. But they do. And even scarier are the moments when happiness is so encompassing that you wonder, if you speak of it, will it all disappear, or will others hate you for being happy?

We need those two, four, six women in our lives who can take it all in and give it right back. The girls who will always support, scale that wall, even if it means breaking a nail or rolling an ankle, and who will always, always be honest. Because honesty is the key. It's what sets us apart from most boys. No man bashing here; I love my guys, but we, as women, have this gift of truth that comes with the X chromosome. It's why we cry at weddings and births and kindergarten registration. Our authenticity shows in every emotional situation. We are rather horrible liars. We're nurturers and nurses and nanas. We see through the B.S. and give what's needed even if it's not asked for. The truth is emotion, and we girls have got it in droves.

But at some point, we stopped letting our emotions lead us to the women we need.

Was it when we got married? Had kids? Turned forty? Lost a parent? Or did it come when we started to hold back what we really felt and stopped sharing the stories that connected us to one another? Those girlfriends are out there, and most of us *are* that friend who just got lost along the way. Everything we are missing from our tribe right now, we can get back, as long as we're willing to give it in return. I know it's hard and it's so much easier to cocoon and isolate because we think that's what keeps us safe from rejection and disappointment. But does it really? One day when the job is done, the kids are grown, the pace slowed, we will really need those girlfriends to help us make sense of who we are apart from all the chaos.

Oh girl, I don't mean that female relationships are easy. They aren't. As complex as we are, these friendships can be some of the most difficult parts of our sentimental navigation. Our emotions often sway like the wind, especially when we are under extreme stress. This is nothing to be ashamed of, but to observe with acceptance. And so, we need to give each other room to make mistakes within our relationships.

I will be the first to raise my hand and say I am not the easiest woman to be friends with. I am awesome at serving others. I will give unyieldingly to every woman around me. I send text messages checking in and meals when times are tough (I promise I won't prepare them). You will always get a birthday card and a phone call. And year after year I'll come back to remind you of your worth even if I haven't heard from you in months. Somehow despite my schedule, the Lord always opens me up to help others. But as soon as I start to need you, things get hard.

Maybe you are the giver in the relationship, and you automatically assume everyone else gives as much as you do, and then get your feelings hurt when they don't. I'm a needy friend. Let's just say it like it is, I'm needy in general. I expect a lot. Perhaps you are too. Raise your hand with pride! You aren't alone. We all have highs and lows. We want our friends to fix us even though we know they can't, and you want to fix them too. Yes, we can be total train wrecks in so many ways, but that doesn't mean we don't try.

For decades I used to think I just wasn't worthy. I'd question why I was always the one giving in the relationship and why I would constantly find these people who couldn't give back. I've learned it's because that's where the Lord needs me. It's where He needs you. He needs us to lead others and be the friend they can open up to and lean on. Even if they walk away after they heal. He has made us strong enough to hold others up and when we begin to sway, *He* will do the same for us. Neediness isn't actually weakness at all but a strength. Close friendships are made stronger by constant presence. As soon as you shed that ego and give in to be the person who is always calling and always planning, you are freed up to serve.

It's taken time, and a lot of soul searching but I found my dream team. Those girls who I can always rely on. Even a few just like me, who constantly surprise me with their desire to serve me so selflessly. And oh, how these women have saved me over and over. You, sweet girl, need to find your haven. As easy as it is to hibernate in your sorrow during this wait, you will get through it with so many more pockets of joy if you work at finding another to share with.

We need people. We need girlfriends, sisters, mothers. We need each other. We can't heal and move on without the help of others. So next time you feel that hole, or wonder where your tribe is, look inside. Figure out how you can help someone else. Reach out to another mother, be vulnerable. Let it be messy so that together you can create something beautiful.

———————⚓———————

Don't Wait: find your girlfriend. Maybe it's one you have lost touch with. Possibly it's someone who has asked you to a drink or coffee, but you've always said no for one reason or another. Perhaps it's a woman in your life who has always been there, but you've taken her for granted. There are those times when it seems impossible to meet people but that's when you need to get even deeper into hearing where the Lord is pushing you. Start saying yes to invitations no matter how exhausted by this pain you feel. You need her. And sister, she needs you too. Today: call or text three women, open yourself up.

———————✢———————

When I'm in a waiting period I try to view it more as a resting period. Rest is positive—to wait is negative. Even the term "rest up" sounds positive. Wait "weighted down" (same words when spoken). The in-between period is meant to recharge, prep time for what is going to come. I try to rest and visualize and actually to start to be grateful before the next event even happens. Even if I don't know what is next or, what decision should be made.

—*Karen*

18

BUY NOW

Are we really doing this?
Yes! I'm hitting buy now.
Eeeek, OMG, I can't believe we are doing it.
I know! Go Us!
Done.
We're going to Miami!!!!

t was no small miracle. A year of planning to get away finally realized in a three-hour text chain of second guessing, doubts, fears, and eventually action.

I had been trying to get Chelsea out of town for a girls' weekend for ages. She needed it. Needed a break from being the giver, the caretaker, the mom, wife, cruise director for her entire family. I recognized that in her, but it was really just a mirror reflection of me.

I had never gone away with just girlfriends. I vacationed all the time, it was my love language, but it was always with my family. I couldn't bear to leave them, and it hurt me to think of taking a plane without them. But I knew I needed it. Mommy-ing was my favorite job, but I needed a break. I needed rest after ten years of full-time working and parenting.

But that made me feel selfish. Made me ask why I should get a break. It also made me scared. How would my husband and three kids survive without me?

Money, scheduling, fear, all of it kept us from planning a trip, but this one day, I did it. I worked past the chaos and doubts for just long enough to buy nonrefundable plane tickets. I let go and let God.

What my friends and I discovered in the next six weeks was the anticipation of those fifty-two hours away was as valuable as the days themselves. Our party of two quickly grew to six, with a couple of the women complete surprises and near strangers to us. But each time another woman heard about our upcoming trip and asked if she could go along, we decided that God wasn't making any mistakes here; if that girl needed to be on this trip, He would put her there regardless of our trepidation.

In the days leading up we started a text chain and we swapped ideas on where to go and what to see and, most importantly where to eat. Each time we saw one another in passing at work or in town, we would squeal with delight and recite the remaining days or hours until takeoff. Our friendships blossomed in ways they can only do when you experience something thrilling and special with another human being.

The trip itself was exactly what we needed. We laughed, we cried, one girl even got sick, but to her defense she usually only has one glass of red wine and us mamas were downing fancy drinks like it was our *job*. I still carry a picture on my phone of our little puker looking gorgeous and smiling (only she looks beautiful after heaving) and her best friend hysterically laughing next to her. We shopped and ate at amazing restaurants. We danced our hearts out and shared stories of our kids and husbands and our dreams and worries. We all agreed the trip was exactly what we needed and not long enough, but we also knew deep down had it been any longer it wouldn't have happened.

We returned home happily exhausted and vowed to do our next trip somewhere that involved detox, yoga, and profession-al-level napping. We walked into our homes to little ones we missed and hugs that were even sweeter because of the absence. Our eyes had more of a softness for our spouses and gratitude for the village that it took to care of the kids, house, and job while we were gone. The house might not have been perfectly clean, and the dog's food bowl may have been a bit bare, but overall everyone survived without us. But maybe that was part of the fear? If they could live without us, where was our worth? But we could see the need in our families' eyes, and for the first time in a long time it didn't feel like neediness, it just felt like the love we sometimes overlooked when looking after *it all*.

Our less than three days away was a blast, but how it changed us in the weeks before and after is what impacted us most. The friendships that became closer, the way we found ourselves again, and the renewed passion for our families that can only come from taking a chance and taking some time for yourself for a few days.

These days, we have dinner whenever one of us is in town, and we still use our text chain as a forum for our accomplishments and defeats. We followed our fifty-two hours with a twenty-four-hour getaway a few months later and we now have a girl's trip on the books at least two times a year. It's not always easy to find the time or money, and the longer we go in between the easier it can be to fall back into second guessing, but we do it. All it really takes is one girlfriend, two nights, and the courage to hit "buy now."

―――――― ⚘ ――――――

Don't Wait:

- *Don't think too long.* Scan your calendar a few months out, find at least two nights, and book the trip. The more time that passes from idea to booking, the more likely you are to find a reason to change your mind. Trust, girlfriend; you need to trust that the Lord has a good plan and a reason for you to get away for a few days. Don't overthink it or let fear of the "what ifs" get in the way. Just book the trip.
- *Designate a treasurer.* This is brilliant. Choose one girl to pay for everything you will be splitting. Hotel, Ubers, meals—everything. She's the keeper of all the receipts and bills (and hopefully sees the benefit this will be if she's using a rewards credit card) and at the end of the trip she divides the total and everyone Venmos! This was perhaps one of the highlights of our first trip. No stress, no splitting checks, no carrying cash! What a blessing this system has been for our relaxation factor.
- *Start a countdown clock.* This helps you reap the benefits of anticipation. Think about advent calendars and Christmas and crossing days off before summer vacation. Each morning it gives you something to wake up and be excited about. I use the app Countdown on my phone.

These days I make a countdown for everything from vacations to date nights.

- *Create a text or email chain.* This is a great place to swap ideas on where to go and build an itinerary. It also helps build that relationship before you leave.

- *Pack light.* For the love of baby Jesus, don't overpack. I don't care where you are headed, you do not need more than two pairs of shoes for a long weekend. Less is more, and girl, you know you are going to shop, so leave some space to spare. If hair tools and toiletries are your downfall, divvy up who is bringing what and share. The good news is if you forget something or need more there are these things called stores everywhere. No more than a small carryon and a nice size purse (or backpack with a purse packed to use when you get there). Trust me, you will not want to be wasting time with luggage when you only have a couple days.

Waiting for something but I'm not sure what. My kids are now older, I have two in college and one in high school, but he is almost gone too. I guess I'm waiting to see what's next. My life has revolved around my kids for so long. And I loved that time. But what happens next? It's not retirement. But it's not just mothering. It's like I'm stopped, but it's not over. There is more to my life, but I don't know what it is. I'm waiting for what is next.

—Bernadette

19

RIGHT NOW

"You are perfectly suited to *not* be a missionary." He laughed at me over the phone.

"Gee thanks," I responded in jest.

"You would last about four days and they would ask you to go home." His laughing is louder now, really full of tickled amusement. Belly laughing, if you will.

I can see what he means, envision myself having a breakdown over not coming in under budget and ahead of schedule in some third world country while I'm just meant to be helping out. The man on the other end of the line is J.R., my spiritual advisor. Think of him as a cross between a life coach and therapist with a whole lot of Jesus in the mix. Exactly what we all need in our lives. He's a short Irish father of three in his fifties who only wears black, drives an old Cadillac, and surfs in jeans. I say that last one because despite the fact that he lived in southern California and I've seen his surfboard, I've never known the guy to wear anything but long pants and a black blazer. We have an ongoing social media battle about my desire to live my life in swimwear and his certainty that the world is a better place when you wear long sleeves. What hair he has left is red, and he cusses like a sailor. He is a pastor. True story: a former news producer and pastor to the porn stars, whose purpose in life is to nurture Christians. He has saved me, truly saved me, over the last decade plus.

The conversation about being a missionary has come up because I am just so sick of myself. Really, I'm exhausting. The head racing, constant catastrophizing, never satisfied, over achieving, horrible at cooking—that one isn't important, it's just my truth—waiting for the other shoe to drop, self. No matter how far I've come, what I have overcome, or how successful I am, I just can't just stop and enjoy. I'm always waiting for what horrible thing that's coming next. I threaten to get rid of all my earthly possessions, quit my job, and move to Uganda.

J.R. urges me to rethink.

"This place of turmoil is exactly where you need to be," he says.

Such a time as this. Sound familiar? I have already dedicated my life to service, by bearing my soul and, in J.R.'s words, "being a damn good witness." He isn't at all surprised by the constant hop from one wait to the next, one struggle to another, because with each one I learn to be a stronger soldier for Christ, and I absorb one more story to pour out on someone in need.

Scaling it all back and getting rid of everything around us isn't going to keep us from running into roadblocks. Life will continue to happen whether you live on a fifty-acre estate or in a yurt in Laos. (Do they have yurts in Laos? No matter, it sounds pretty simple, but then again maybe not.) In many of us there will always be a light shining on what isn't right as opposed to focusing on all that is. (The yurt is strong, the weather good, but oh yeah, *you're in a yurt in Laos.*)

He tells me to stop. Just stop. Take a breath and realize I'm okay right now.

You are okay right now.

You *are* okay right now.

You are somewhere reading these words and, in this moment, you are okay. We are not talking about a week from now, an hour from now, even the next minute. We're talking about right now. And right now, you are okay. When you are struggling with waking up every morning gripped by fear and worry, stop and repeat: you are okay right now. Whether your worry is a result of big scary looming trauma, or just the everyday stuff that seems to leave us overwhelmed—kids in college, aging parents, gray roots, laundry...stop me please.

Stop.

You are okay right now.

Boil it down to this second. Wake up, breathe deep, look around, and accept that right now is okay. As I was two years into working through my fears, and still struggling with the same demons in my life, J.R. finally told me to pinch myself. Yep, the soft stuff wasn't working, we were resorting to violence. This girl was messed up! But a blessed, beautiful mess I am. For me, it's needing to get over the loss in the past so I can enjoy the present. God has brought me through all the crap.

All. The. Crap.

And I am here, stronger, and more blessed as a result. But I hate that. Because I hate what I went through. Hate what I am still going through. I continue to feel the fall. The moment the worst happens. The bracing for the next punch. It's muscle memory. PTSD. Fear. Call it what you will, it's what keeps me from believing it's all okay. Because it's not the bad thing that I'm really afraid of, it's that I don't want to go through the pain. We are programmed to avoid pain. We have this promise in our God that we will have eternal life, He will not leave us or forsake us, but that doesn't mean we don't have to get to the other side of tough times. Really tough times. So, while I believe that it will all turn out for His good, I hate going through the pain. I will avoid pain at all costs when what I really need to be doing is walking in it with my head held high and my hand encased in my Lord's.

But I am okay, right now. And you are okay, right now.

Pinch.

I get that you may be in the battle. Not waiting for the next one, but in it now. You are gripped with anxiety because your spouse is no longer next to you, your child is in the hospital miles away, the job you felt defined you is now gone, or the deep breath you are trying to take is strangled by disease. Nothing feels okay right now. But it is.

It's okay to wake up in fear.

It's okay to be sick of the way you feel.

It's okay to not know how to get over your past, or dread your future.

Just remember: it's okay right now. You are okay, but you can't do this alone. Just as we need people, we need professionals. Therapists, doctors, a team. Please, accept that we are not a solitary species. We need the expertise of others.

The majority of my extended family is pretty far away. They will call and innocently ask how everyone is doing. I'll be honest in my, "Great!" because it's the truth. We are flawed and fabulous. I'll often follow up with a rundown of the week's events. Imagine me heaving out a twenty-pound scroll, the end of it dropping to the ground and rolling two hundred yards down the driveway. We're often that kind of busy up in here. "We're great, busy but great! Soccer, cheer, art class and of course everyone is in therapy—yesterday for Grace, tomorrow for Georgia, Dan on Thursday, but we're good!"

It's not something most people include in innocent conversation, but I feel like it's so important to talk about. Just as we aren't to be ashamed of adoption or miscarriage or addiction we need to work to make therapy less of a stigma. I'm not ashamed. In fact, I feel like it's a win for team Lindquist! Therapy is a safety net for my kids and a life vest for me. Not everyone sees the benefit of voicing their pain; the first time my middle child went to therapy she decided she wasn't going to go back.

"Mom, I went in perfectly happy and by the time I left I was crying."

"Yeah, well that's kind of the point kiddo."

Therapy isn't painless and often in the beginning it feels worse, but that is growth my friend, that's you healing. Georgia is now a big fan. I let her lead because she is strong enough, and she eventually asked to go back. That little girl is an anomaly, and especially with adolescents you may have to drag them kicking and screaming, but it's so much easier to lead by example from the time they are little. Just as it's perfectly normal to be a mixed-race family, have a mom that's on TV, or say a prayer before dinner, therapy is completely common, and they have seen us going since they were babies. It's not scary. It's necessary.

The problem for me has always been finding the right therapist. I know I'm a special case, I can talk all day about the cobweb
of crazy, but what I need is someone to give me tangible advice on
how to clean it up! And don't you dare come to me with solutions
unless they contain a big spoonful of Jesus. That's why having a
spiritual advisor works for me. He gives actual ideas on how to
change course instead of just asking me how I feel. I don't know
how I feel half the time! And most importantly, we discuss all of
this bookended in prayer.

The key is honesty. You can find the perfect match, but if you
aren't telling the truth and opening up all the dark parts you have
kept hidden, you aren't going to benefit. This doesn't even have to
be done with a professional in the beginning. Often, it's easier and
less scary to talk it out with a stranger who listens for a living, but
it can be done with a friend or a support group. Start by just being
authentic with those around you. Admit to the marital problems
when you are on the phone with your girlfriend. Talk about your
fears of inadequacy with your sister. Connect with a bible study.

This is another area where you may need to try a few before
you find the right study. Find women who are in your age group or
look for a group at a local church that speaks to what you are going
through. Even start one if you can't find the right fit. I run a bible
study out of my home twice a month. I created it because I couldn't
find a group in my area that met at a time that worked *and* was full
of women like me. This gathering at my home can sometimes be
twenty people and sometimes just two. I try really hard not to get
my feelings hurt when everyone cancels at the last minute. It's just
my own ego, and God is teaching me through the discomfort. I
know no matter who shows up God is creating the exact environ-

ment He needs. He is opening me up to be a safe place for whomever arrives. And just as importantly, He is giving me other women I can ask for help. I need them as much as they need me.

If you are a widow or going through a divorce or lost a child, get to a support group. If you're battling cancer or illness, use the hospital resources to find others in the same situation. If addiction is part of your waiting period, get your bum to an Alcoholics Anonymous meeting, or an Al-Anon meeting. Then stick with it. Don't just go once, go back again and again and get the support you need. I know it's scary, I know it can make you feel so vulnerable and like a failure, I know because I have been there. I sat in that room with other souls broken like me and I cried my way through it, but it worked. Just tell the truth. Open up and find others who can help.

You can do this alone. But probably not well. And honestly girl, why would you? Nothing you reveal is as horrible as you are making it out to be in your mind. Others are going through exactly what you are. Let that commonality help you heal. You get a trainer to help you get in shape, consult a diet plan to lose weight, find a financial advisor to plan your future, why would you not get help for the most important aspect of your life: your mental health? Asking for help doesn't mean anything is wrong with you, in fact it means you are getting better and becoming smarter.

Don't Wait:

- What in this moment is okay? Is it your family, your job, your home? Maybe you need to think smaller—the weather, the book in your hands, the color of the walls in your room? Hold on to that right now. Don't focus on what is coming or what's behind but embrace what is positive now. And write this down: I am okay right now. Meditate on it, memorize it, sing it if you need to, just don't forget you *are* okay.

- Now find help. A therapist, a spiritual advisor, a pastor to talk to. Get to a group, or even tell a friend. Make yourself a priority. You need to let it out, just get it out, and move on. How is up to you. A Google search will work, a look at your benefits web page at work, or even use my spiritual advisor, his name and number are literally in the back of the book. Just, oh babe, don't do this alone. Right now, write down three ideas for support. People or groups or professionals.

_____

_____

_____

- Now follow through. Finding a therapist isn't always easy, and this is another area of your life where you could easily make excuses. First, get rid of your ego and accept you need help and can't do it alone. Next, understand that it may take you a few different people before you find the one that works for you. If you talk to a therapist and you don't feel better or at least like that you are growing after that first session, go and find another one. You have to put in the work. I've had more than a handful of therapists that just didn't click. And yes, it was a pain in the rear to go through all the insurance stuff and scheduling and then have to do it all over again and again until I found someone who worked. But it was worth it, and so freaking necessary. If your child was sick, you would go to doctor after doctor until you found the right one. You are our Lord's child; treat yourself as such and get the help you need.

———————✞———————

Spiritual Direction takes the guesswork out of a relationship with God. It centers in the space between two people seeking the voice and movement of God. One person listening intently as another narrates the current season of life. Both people knowing God sits at the center of the words and emotions. Spiritual direction seeks the intimacy of community, giving power to carry each other's burdens. A good spiritual director will help you hear your voice and identify true self. A good spiritual director will not make things easy. And lastly, a good spiritual director never steps into the spotlight that holds the Divine.

—*Spiritual Director, J.R. Mahon*

REST

Teach me to let go.

20

CHILDLIKE

A woman from work always asks how my babies are doing. Every day I pass by her office she kindly repeats her inquiry with a smile. Over the years, my babies have grown from toddlers to little girls, and eventually their baby brother came along, and I started over. Gratefully, I respond, "they are great," and "beautiful," and "I'm so lucky," because no matter how hard parenting can be, that is always the big picture truth.

One cold winter day I paused for a second and thought about my answer as opposed to just giving my automatic response. I thought through the morning, just hours before, and our cuddles on the couch after they woke up. I remember I didn't want to break contact with my three favorite humans. My colleague stopped, let me finish, and with such love in her eyes said,

"That thing, that yearning to hold them, oh dear, it never leaves." Her twenty-two-year-old daughter was home for a few days, and she told me how she would pull her close and inhale the scent of her.

For a brief moment, I thought that action sort of odd. A grown woman smelling another. But when I got home, I picked up the baby and instinctively pulled him to my face and inhaled that luscious scent that meant more to me than air. I could stay there all day, just wrapped in him. When my daughters got home, one by one, I cuddled them tight and buried my nose in their messy hair and breathed in the sweet, earthy smell of my little girls. I understood what my friend was saying. I never want to stop. I can see myself wanting to inhabit my daughters' space even one day when they are bigger than me. I will always want to hold them because they are my children.

———————————✣———————————

I think we forget what it is to feel nurtured like a child: to be held and cradled and to be devoured by love. But that's what our heavenly Father yearns to do every day. He wants to comfort us and hold us and drink us in. That love I feel for the three amazing people I get to raise is the same love He feels for each and every one of His children. Encompassing, unwavering, irrational. Even when we are lost. Even when we forget about his love. Even when we have left Him behind. He will never stop loving us and wanting to bring us home and hold us like a child.

Take a look at Luke 15:11–32. The father in the story of the prodigal son suffered so much. He saw his younger son leave, knowing the disappointments, rejections, and abuses facing him. He saw his older son become angry and bitter yet was unable to offer him affection and support. A large part of the father's life had been spent waiting. He could not force his younger son to come home or his older son to let go of his resentments. Only they themselves could take the initiative to return. During these long years of waiting, the father cried many tears and died many deaths.

Imagine what that was like for the father.

Some of you are in this waiting for your child and it is tearing you apart. The father in this story was emptied out by suffering. He was broken. But that emptiness, that brokenness created a place of welcome. It opened him up to an all-encompassing love for his sons when the time of their return came. We are all called to become like that father, to wait on the Lord and allow ourselves to be emptied so God can fill us up. But we are also reminded in this story that we are the prodigal son. We stray from our daddy so often in our pain. Yet, He will never give up on us. He is forever in us. Always.

We are only as happy as our most miserable child. You've heard that saying. Oh, how true it is. I have to believe our father feels the same. Like the prodigal father, when one of our children is astray or in pain, we are as well.

When I'm feeling lost, I put myself back in the position of my Father's child. I imagine how He longs to comfort me, as I so long to comfort my own kids. Some days I only get a moment of closeness before my child pulls away in favor of the next activity. But some days, if she is having a rough day, she will cuddle in close and stay with me for hours. When he is sick, he will grab a blanket and use me as pillow and beg me not to go. These are the times I love the most. They need no one but me, they trust me completely, and desire to be nowhere but right in that moment.

When is the last time you allowed yourself to release like that? To let go of control and surrender? There is always some action to be taken, a move to make that takes us out of His loving embrace. I know, we are adults, we have the weight of the world on our shoulders. We have responsibilities and people we are responsible for, but we are still His children. Just as I pray my kids will always collapse into my embrace when they are grown and let me inhale their struggles and hold them up when they are weak, He is longing for us to do the same. To stop and be like a child again.

Take a moment, return in your heart, to your parents' embrace. If your childhood wasn't full of affection and comfort, then imagine a time that was. How does it feel? What do you hear? How do you breathe? What do you see? Release your shoulders and exhale into that love. Spend a minute, five minutes, thirty minutes, if you can, and return to the younger version of you. The one that craved cuddling and compassion and trusted that mom and dad would fix it all. Now allow that parent to be your Lord. Feel His perfect presence, His impenetrable security. Because He is waiting. He will never leave. He will always be there wanting to pull you in and smell your head and never let go. No matter how old you are, you will always be His child. Let your guard down and let Him be your papa.

Feel His perfect presence, His impenetrable security.

Don't Wait: take a moment and put yourself in this place.

He is sitting next to you, closely, head slightly bowed and a small smile on His holy lips.

"Sweet girl," He whispers, "You're okay. Everyone you love is okay. Please stop wasting these precious moments in fear and worry. This is a fruitless mental obstacle course. Trust me. I love you so much and I will carry you through every physical, emotional, and financial battle."

You look at Him, tears in your eyes. Relief, embarrassment. He reaches His arm around you, a side hug, then as you melt, tension and resistance disappear, He leans all the way in and holds you close, both arms wrapped around you in an encompassing embrace.

"Oh, my baby girl, you are such a good daughter. I am so proud of you. It's okay, I'm here, you don't need to carry all of this. I am much stronger. It will all be okay, I promise."

You exhale and let it all go.

Now let *it all go*. It's a physical movement. You can feel the weight drip off. All the worry, all the sadness, all the fear leaves your body. At least for a moment. And that moment is everything. I'm not saying it won't return—the pressure and paralyzing unknown. But if you can sit every day, multiple times a day even, and let it go and give it all to Him, you can feel relief.

PRAYER TO YOUR FATHER

> *Lord, please come to me. I'm here. I'm your servant, I'm your child and I'm scared. Please put your arms around me and tell me it will all be okay. Fix this thing that feels broken inside me. This part of me that allows fear more room than you. This worry consumes me, and I want to be consumed by your love instead. I know you are bigger than this. I*

know in a second my reality could change because you are almighty. You parted the sea twice! You can take a breath, and this will all change. Yet, I tremble in fear, not of you, but of the things of this world. Why Lord, why? Why am I having such a hard time finding rest in your word? Your promise? Your love?

Oh, my father, how I love you so much. My whole body longs to fall on you, collapse into your strength. Hold me up. Make all this earthly pain vanish with the sound of your voice. And it can, it will, if I just let it. Perhaps I am the barrier between us. You are here waiting for me to give up and give in. I do Lord, I do! Please take this struggle. All of it is too much for me. I want only your glory to greet me each morning, not the wicked lies of this world that torment my mind and my heart. Clear the concern, erase my attempts to control.

Please Lord, meet me. Your power is awesome, and I need you. When my thoughts start to drift to "what if," lead me back to, "my God." When it seems impossible for me, remind me of you. I love you Lord and thank you for the abundance you have already placed in my life. I am not worthy of a thing, except your love; but I am so grateful you have rained down such blessings on your child. Help me to remember every impossible situation and remarkable outcome instead of focusing on what you have yet to conquer for me.

Yet—*that is the word.*

You will conquer this, even if the big demon is simply my own mind.

21

REMEMBER

et's do a little exercise together. Not the kind that works your body, though I hope you have made the time for that today; this one works your heart and mind. Get comfortable, minimize distractions, and give yourself three minutes to remember. Go back into your memories to a time when God came through in a huge way. A situation that you lost sleep over, cried over, couldn't see your way out of where He, in the end, worked miracles. There have most likely been more than a few. I'm not asking you for small things, like finding a lost wedding ring after a week (been there) or that time you drove home after having had more than you probably should have to drink (yep, not proud of it, but me too). While not insignificant, those aren't the situations I'm talking about. I want the time the scan came back with the cancer gone, the lawsuit settled, or the son that was so lost to addiction finally agreeing to rehab. A time that had a moment. One huge moment when everything worked out and *it was good*.

There have been quite a few times in my life where God has provided when I felt it was hopeless. It is never hopeless. Never.

Many of the jobs I've had in my life have been nearly unattainable. Nine thousand people auditioned for the position I wanted, and I was one of two hired. How's that for coming through? Job loss has also been a huge part of my family's life, and each time the Lord works it out or at least gives us the learnings from our directional shift. Getting pregnant and carrying a healthy child to term was a miracle in itself. And each adoption held at least one moment where a hurdle was crossed or a clock ran out, and we made it through.

I wrote about one moment in my book, *5 Months Apart: A Story of Infertility, Faith and Grace.* The birth father for our first daughter had decided not to sign the paperwork, and we were close to losing this child we already loved. Then, miraculously, he changed his mind. It all happened in one moment on the phone.

> *The day Marisol called to say that Alex signed the papers, I felt relief as intense and physical as childbirth…I wanted to reach through the phone and hug her until she turned blue. Relief rose from my toes to my eyes, and I sobbed happy tears. I had prayed to God so many times in the past few years, but this time, I fell violently to my knees. I whispered thank you, thank you, thank you, until my folded hands were drenched in tears. My knees became my preferred spot from that moment on. Submitting to Him. Glorifying Him. Rejoicing in Him. He had done this.*[4]

---

[4] Lindquist, Kerstin (2017). *5 Months Apart: A Story of Infertility, Faith and Grace.* Elk Lake.

That was a physical release for me. All that energy caught up and finally washed out with that one phone call. There's no feeling like it. What about for you? Are you there? Can you remember? Where were you? Visualize the room. Was it bright or dark? Was the temperature warm or cold? Who was with you? What could you smell or taste? Were you seated or standing? Close your eyes and go back. What happened when the news came? When your mind clicked, and you realized it was all going to be okay. Something you had prayed for without ceasing was finally realized. The weight was lifted, you were saved. What did you do? Did you cry or laugh? Did you fall to your knees and thank the Lord? Did you even realize it was the Lord's work at the time or did you forget him in your gratitude? How was your heartbeat, your color? Were there goosebumps or chills, or did the relief come so immediately that you quickly fell asleep after too many restless, anxiety-filled nights?

Now, as the euphoria drifted, did any part of you think perhaps you should have trusted Him more because of course, this was something He would take care of? It's easy to remember in detail the pain in the hard times, but it's often hard to recall as vividly the way you felt when it was over and everything turned out alright. Sit there for a moment and feel it. He fixed it, He made it okay, He saved you. He always will. It may not be the solution you prayed for, but often it is. And regardless, He is not going to let you down. Instead of listing the times it didn't work out, write down all the times it did! And dwell there, sister. In fact, write down three descriptive words that can get you back to that moment. For me those words are: relief, gratitude, and weeping. They were such happy tears and I can feel them still. I was so in love with my God at that moment, and those three words get me back there at any time. Use your three words to recall what you felt. Memorize them, and when you are so stuck on what is wrong, go back to that time it was so right. Especially when it seems like this current waiting period is impossible, visualize the time He came through in the past and trust He will again.

> *It's easy to remember in detail the pain in the hard times, but it's often hard to recall as vividly the way you felt when it was over and everything turned out alright.*

Yeah, sounds easy enough, right? I know it's not. Even as I write this, my family is drowning in our favorite kind (insert eye roll) of waiting period, a financial one. It brings me to tears every time I think about it, and each time I try to imagine how it's going to all work out, I spiral into a hopeless pity party. No mariachi and guacamole, this is a true *pity* party. All this torture despite the fact that He has gotten us through these situations before. Why can't I just remember!?

I'm the caretaker in the family, the planner, the one who does the bills and makes the budget. Each time we end up in a money quandary I feel like a failure. Finances are one of those places where people secretly judge. Like sex. Everyone has it in their life to some extent, but no one wants to talk about it for fear of comparison. Especially for Christians it can feel dirty and be full of anxiety, guilt, and shame. (Both money and sex, we Christians can use some major therapy in those areas.) We know that money isn't the most important thing and that God will provide, and we know the whole camel and the eye of the needle story we learned at age twelve, but it's hard to live that out. When we voice our money concerns, it's often met with condescending phrases about being thankful for what you have, but few of the people who say those words are giving away all their possessions and serving the poor. And if you are, then you, yes *you*, can judge. I welcome it, because you have earned it, and you will probably do it with a loving heart. The thing is, we all need money, and God wants to bless us. Despite living nearly my entire adult life paycheck to paycheck, I know the Lord wants to pour out all the riches of heaven. And He has. Maybe not in the abundance I had hoped for, but He always provides. Which is why no matter how tough it gets we never stop tithing. Never. Another non-negotiable. Even in this moment now, where I don't know how we are going to afford this life we've created, and it breaks my heart to tell my kids no, God gets His first. He will always provide more, as long as we are faithful in what he has already given us. I know this is true. We haven't had to sell a child (yet). There's been times when I've had to sell all I could find on eBay, once we had to sell a car, and we've even sadly lost more than one home, but we are still standing. And we are filled with overflowing love and abundance way beyond our bank account.

Maybe your wait right now is a financial one. Don't be ashamed. It may seem trivial at times when you have people around you battling disease and death, but this is your trial right now and it's okay for you to feel this stress at these times. Just remember. Remember when He came through. Even though we did end up losing our savings as well as our baby, and even after we did lose our home to a short sale, we eventually rose again. We expanded our family, we built up our savings, we found another home. Our pain in those hard times wasn't diminished, but there was always a moment when it worked out.

Live in that moment.

Breathe it in.

Don't Wait:

- Take three minutes in silence to remember. Use the question prompts in the above chapter to get your mind back into that space. Sit up straight, knees above your ankles, like you did in school or church. Relax your hands and close your eyes. If your mind drifts too frequently with closed eyes, then open them and focus on one spot.
- Now pick the three descriptive words from that memory and use them as a reminder. Put them in a journal, write them as a note on your computer or your phone. Write them on sticky notes and put them on your mirror.

Words that have some significance to me in these moments are:

Relief
Gratitude
Weeping
Exhale
Joy
Release
Awakening
Weightlessness

Happiness
Rejoicing
Thankfulness
Realization
Perfection

When the anxiety rises, say your three words, close your eyes, and go back to that room. That moment. I want you to have all those feelings. Soon it will be easier to remember the pleasure than it is the pain.

———————❦———————

We had the longest wait when we were getting our business going. I had to put all my dreams of owning a home and car and all the "grown up stuff" on hold, even getting married and having kids was shifted, because we needed to wait and build our foundation.

I had these friends all getting their careers going and moving on with next life steps and I was so discouraged at times wondering if my day for those things I so wanted would happen. I questioned if waiting for this dream was the right thing to do, because what if we failed and I missed out on all I had been waiting for. Waiting and being patient, being disciplined and making certain sacrifices along the way was necessary for us for a long-term return. It just wasn't easy.

—Ally

22

LETTER TO MY YOUNGER SELF

Dear Kerstin,

Hey there, seventeen; you're pretty awesome, you know that? No really. Now that we have daughters of our own, I can see it's a miracle mom let us out of the house and gave us such freedom. There is so much to fear for a girl your age. So many mistakes that can be made and dangers that lurk and you haven't just survived, you've thrived. Keep your faith and trust your gut and you will be fine. (Especially when you are travelling through Spain—don't go into that bathroom in the nightclub!)

I'm extremely proud of you for learning the value of work so young. Those jobs you've had through high school will help you mature and be so successful when you get older. I know how much you love being a lifeguard, love the sun, love the boys (things you will always love) but sweetie, wear sunscreen! We're going to pay for that baby oil at forty.

Bravo for getting into and nailing college. This will be one of the best times of your life, but you don't have to go to the most expensive college to get that experience. Mom wants the best for you, but we will also be paying for that when we're forty so maybe choose one a little less pricey. It will still be great; YOU will make it great. Just take Spanish not French, please. In all other matters, listen to mom and take her advice. Sometimes she holds on a little too tight, but there is going to come a time, way too soon, that you would give anything for her to be there to hold you again.

Oh, look at you, twenty-seven. Get out right!? Already married for two years. There's a lesson here, doll: you can try to drive your future, but God's plan is always better. I know you didn't expect to find the love of your life so young, but this move to get married so quickly after meeting Dan will be one of the best decisions you will ever make. He's a one-of-a-kind, godly guy. No matter how hard life gets, and girl, you are in for a very rough ride at times, he will always adore you and be your best friend. This part of your story came easy. And I want you to remember that, because this relationship will get very hard down the road. But things can and will work out for you.

A couple things will help you in the next ten years. Don't do that funky loan. Put twenty or even thirty percent down. In fact, save as much as you can so you can pay in cash whenever possible! That being said, get the convertible VW Beetle. It seems like a luxury as opposed to the logical sedan, but that car will bring you so much joy. And please, oh please never delay joy. There is too much suffering, so find the happiness. Get used to making hard decisions. Moving will be a common part of your life. Lots of changes, and I know change is hard for you, but there is a fine line between fear and excitement. Look at each season as exciting. Don't be afraid. God's got you. Don't get too attached to things. Building, acquiring, buying. These things are not your worth. You will have to say goodbye often and they do not define you. But people, people do. Get attached, fall in love, make tremendous friends. Leaving them will always be hard, and it may seem easier to not become attached so you don't have to go through the pain of loss, but you will be made complete by the people you let in. People are worth it, and your friends are worth the pain.

You will finally stop struggling with those last ten pounds after you turn forty. The answer is broccoli. Yep, broccoli for every meal, and cut out the cheese. Once you do, you will finally feel better about yourself and stop battling your weight. Oh, and tequila. Good sipping tequila. No fruity drinks, less wine. Sipping tequila will not leave you hung over and won't add the pounds. And get enough sleep! Seven and a half hours at least. Guard your sleep. Dementia and cancer run in your family and you're too important to risk your health. So, go to bed earlier. That way you can also get up earlier and find some quiet time with God. That will change your life too. It will drive away the fear that is going to plague you for the next decade. After you pray, work out. Keep exercising. Those good endorphins will keep you sane and fitness will always be a part of how you support your family.

Now for the family part. It hurts me to write this. It's going to be hard. There is going to be some unbearable loss in your attempt to create a family. If you let it, it will break your marriage, ruin your friendships, and threaten your life. You will survive and let me help you get through; there is overwhelming light on the other side of the darkness. You will be a mother. In fact, the family you have will be bigger and better than you could ever imagine. It just won't come about the way you planned. And that's okay; remember God's plan is better. Don't give up hope no matter how hard it gets. Cling to Dan, don't shut down. Talk about your feelings early. There are so many other women around you who are going through the same thing and there is power and healing in sharing your story. In fact, sounds crazy, but this pain you feel will go on to help and heal thousands. This next decade is when the Lord will allow you to break so you can be used for Him. This is the moment for which you, sweet girl, were created.

You're pushing the big 4-0 and the best is yet to come! And sadly, the worst of your life so far, is also on the way. Yeah, I know, you feel like you made it through so much, how can it get any better or any worse? How will you survive? But you will. By the grace of God, you will. Those little girls who make you feel like you can't breathe through the swell of your heart, aren't the end of your family. There is more! What!? Three!? I know! But you also knew in your heart you never felt you were done with two.

Finish your book. I know it hurts to write, but it will help so many women and, in a way, it will help you heal. You will have the job you always dreamed of, the opportunity to serve those around you, and you will even end up on the *Today* Show! Amazing right?

Money has always been your biggest challenge, and please, oh please, don't let it hold you captive. You feel the weight of the world on your shoulders providing for a family and supporting your husband as he struggles to find his joy, but it's not all on you. Your finances are in God's hand. He will provide. Never stop tithing, giving, and of course praying. Even when it seems like you won't be able to pay the mortgage or buy groceries, I promise you will. Don't lose sleep over things you can't control. God will always, always provide.

Everyone tells you to be so thankful for the hard moments of early motherhood. Be present, don't blink, all that. You have done a great job. You have been so in the moment with those babies. You didn't miss a thing and you have done an amazing job of being a mother. Don't let the guilt get to you. Other moms will always look more pulled together, smarter, prettier, better at baking…but they are just as much of a mess as you are. Grabbing the chardonnay out of the fridge while you give the babies a bath in the kitchen sink is totally acceptable. Motherhood is hard. Cry it out, drink the wine, and ask for help! You have a lot of pride and feel like you should be able to do it all alone, but you can't. And when you finally accept help, you will make some of the best friendships of your life. You thought high school was hard for girlfriends, get ready for grade school moms. It will actually get harder to make strong connections through the next few years of your life, but don't try so hard. If the women around you don't build you up and help you stay close to God, then walk away. A few great friends are better than a dozen mediocre ones.

In fact, walk away often. Say no to things. Guard your time. Only do what makes you truly happy. You've spent so many years building a career you love but the sooner you learn that work is not as important as your family, your health, your joy, the happier you will be. More money isn't worth the time away from the people you love. You'll figure that out in a couple years, and it will bring you such peace.

And go to your twenty-year college reunion. It sounds scary and uncomfortable, but it will bring you closure and remind you of how blessed you were then and now. Those people need you as much as you need them. This sounds like a lot, and I know you are often overwhelmed. That fear will forever threaten to bring you down. But listen to this: at forty, just like everyone said, you start to figure it out. Forty brings peace and contentment. It's not that the struggles stop, in fact they never do. It's not that you are struggling, kiddo, you are just living. You finally learn how to really trust God and navigate the endless trials with grace. Keep yourself in the light of the Lord, girl. Your life will be the stuff of which books are written. You are blessed. And I love you so, so much. Love yourself too.

Xoxo

Your badass self!

———— ✤ ————

Don't Wait:

- Write a letter to yourself. Remind yourself what you have been through and how you survived. Focus on the times when you wish someone would have told you it was all going to work out.
- Now throw in some major self-love. Congratulate, praise, and nurture.
- Place it somewhere you can read it often.
- Write this letter to yourself again every few years as things change.
- Get a pad of sticky notes and reread the letter, underlining major victories. Write down all the times you overcame, or it all worked out when you thought hope was lost. My notes say things like my kids' names, the name of the company I work for, my home, my husband, and so on.

Put these on your vanity or in the back of your planner or somewhere you can constantly be reminded of how God took care of you.

- Every year, go back and write a smaller version of this for the last year. Catalogue your successes and when God came through in a huge way.

- Every week (I usually do Sunday or Monday) go back through your week and write down what went right. Again, recall your successes, and what you accomplished.

———————⚓———————

I waited seventeen years for my beautiful mother to die as she battled breast cancer. Then many more waiting to understand why. We had so much time together yet so little. I went through all of the emotions with God. Sadness, anger, finally acceptance. Years later I was sitting at the kitchen table with my dad and my husband. We had just had a beautiful set of twins and we were embracing not only our complete exhaustion but our complete joy. My father looked at me and said, "You know…this is why she left."

"What do you mean, Daddy?" I replied.

"You and your mom were so close. You were so connected. She knew that in order for you to achieve all of this beauty in your life, that she would have to leave. She was sick and she knew that you would never leave her side. She wanted to watch you fly and all of this beauty you are surrounded with is because of her."

All of a sudden, I felt this complete wave of peace. I finally understood that for all these years I was waiting for this reason, for this answer, I just didn't know that I was waiting. Sometimes, the wait is hidden. Keep waiting. Because it can be so very worth it.

—Mally

IN HIS TIME

"I am the Lord, I will accomplish it quickly in its Time."
Isaiah 60:22 (NIV)

23

PASSAGE OF TIME

The Passages section of *People* magazine haunts me. Every time I hit the mid-point in that popular magazine, my body tightens and my breath quickens. The records of celebrities' weddings, births, and deaths shouldn't have so much power over me, but they do.

As a girl, I was focused on who was getting married. I'd see one of my favorite actors or singers' names pop up and I'd deflate, knowing there was one more hottie to whom I would never be linked. I mean come on, I didn't actually think I was going to stumble across Joey McIntyre one day and he was going to fall madly in love with me, but to my childish defense, I did live outside Los Angeles and I *was* going to be a famous actress, so a girl could dream. Side note: I was obsessed with the New Kids On The Block. Like, I wore all the shirts, collected the comic books, dolls, posters and even authored a newsletter. I still do the iconic dance for my daughters at home as they squeal with embarrassed delight. I cried many a tear over the youngest member of the band because my love was *that* strong. When he went off the market, I died a little.

After I found my own boy band-level hottie and married him in record time, it became the births section that I focused on. By the time I was thirty and deep into infertility, the report that another celebrity my age had given birth would send me into a spiral. I studied the ages at which these women were having babies. If they were older than me, I would reason it could still happen for me. If they were younger, it would confirm I was running out of time.

That self-destructive exercise lasted for over ten years. Every time I went to the nail salon, took a plane, or sat by the beach, I'd open up the glossy pages and allow other peoples' timelines to dictate how I was going to feel about myself. Even after my first two children were born, my comparison became who was having three, or four, and most importantly, that little bold number next to their name that revealed their age. Always concerned time was quickly smothering my dreams.

Now I still find myself looking at the ages of these women having babies and it is nostalgia I feel. A part of me longs to have my babies back, while most of me is thrilled to have what I consider my perfect family and less sleepless nights. These days I look more at the birthdays and compare myself to women my own age. Totally disgusting, and I'm not proud of this act, but it's a truth you probably recognize. The last time I opened the magazine I found myself glancing at the death section. Previously, so concerned with becoming fully immersed in life, I now wonder how I have become so much closer to death. It's not my own I contemplate so much as the passing of those whom I've assumed would always be around. While not part of my family or even friends, so many of the personalities who end up on those pages were staples in my youth and now they are gone. A reminder that we're all moving so fast.

———————✤———————

Time *is* moving so fast. There will be seasons in your life where the wait is truly unknown. Life is happening at record speed and you aren't sure what you should be looking for. There isn't this looming event or struggle, you're just waiting on life. You wonder what comes next. The comparison game in that situation can drive you crazy, and it's not what the good Lord wants for you. Someone else's timeline has no bearing on yours. God is doing His work in you at the pace He knows is best. Isaiah 60:22 says, "I am the Lord, I will accomplish it quickly in its Time." Not your time, not their time, but—

In its time.

If you continue to look around you for where you should be and when, you will miss where you are now.

Someone else's timeline has no bearing on yours.

These are times of rest. You aren't in a period of waiting but a period of rest. You will hit this resting place more than a few times in your life. Before you find your partner. Before the babies come. After the children leave for college. Decades into marriage when things seem to just be coasting along and you aren't sure if that's a good thing or not. The first years of retirement. The end of life.

So often these are times for which we have prepared. There were mountains you had to climb, a finish line you were trying to hit. Now that you made it, you wonder what comes next. We react with planning and filling up with movement and juggling, when what we need is rest.

Rest. Rest is what you need.

Since before I had children, I wanted to be a stay-at-home mom. Granted I had no idea how hard it would be, but I knew I wanted more than anything to be around my kids as much as humanly possible. No job could come close to making me as happy as motherhood. While my career didn't come easy, I was frequently successful. Perhaps having been fulfilled at a job outside the home led me to a want to conquer motherhood. (This anecdote is in no way meant to offend stay-at-home moms. That job is killer. You deserve to be paid a high six figures, get a company car, and paid trips to Hawaii biannually. Most men can't do it and even a majority of women don't have what it takes. Those little humans are often the worst! From the entire country to you, stay-at-home mom, let me say thank you. You are raising the future and we are grateful.) Still, to this day I know I am up for the challenge. And I want it. These kids were so hard to come by, I just don't want to miss a moment. If given the opportunity, I would happily walk away from TV and a public life and stay home and immerse myself in raising the three people I love the most (oh, and serving my husband; yeah, yeah, love you too babe). Yet many of my beloved family members beg to differ. They don't think I have what it takes to stand still.

Leaving a fast-paced career would mean less structure, less hustle. I've been told there is no way I would give up the speed. I get a little defensive on this topic of leaving my job for motherhood. (Shocker—I know, that's so entirely out of character, said with extreme sarcasm.) I ball my fists and dive into a list of reasons why I could and would say goodbye in a second!

Try me. Give me the chance!

But those who kindly reason against me do have a point in one area—I wouldn't slow down. I imagine myself volunteering at all the kid's schools, signing up for every fundraiser, heading the board of something here and something there, choreographing talent shows, cooking for neighbors (No, no, not that one, I am not to be trusted with anything beyond Nutrisystem muffins and broccoli!)—you get the point. Leaving the glamour of TV wouldn't equate to sweatpants (by the way, do people still wear sweatpants? Truly, leggings, joggers, even palazzo pants are so much comfier and still stylish!) and sleeping until noon. But maybe that is the point. I wouldn't be happy leaving my job because that would mean I would have to press the brakes a little. The kids would need some downtime. I couldn't demand action and enforce deadlines like I do in a corporate setting. There would need to be built-in rest. And I don't do rest well.

My spiritual advisor asked me the other day how I was doing in this area.

"I get seven to nine hours of sleep a night," I replied.

He laughed. He does that a lot, apparently my crazy cracks him up. "Not how are you sleeping, but are you resting?"

What is this you speak of? Rest? How can I possibly rest when the house is burning down around me and I am, of course, the only one that can save it.

Oh.

The constant movement isn't doing me any good and isn't serving you either, dear one. We are called to rest. "Return to your rest my soul, for the Lord has been good to you." (Psalm 116:7, NIV) By constantly comparing ourselves to those around us and trying to get to the next chapter, we are skipping over our time of rest. We are givers and lovers and servants and perhaps all you are doing is for His good. But even He will tell you to take a beat. Allow yourself to slow down and feel. That's it, isn't it? You don't stop moving because when you do, you have to *feel*.

We all know those women who are so overscheduled it makes you want to take a nap just thinking about them. Four kids, two travel sports teams each, school treasurer, Girl Scouts leader, alumni president, and a full-time job. When someone asks her to do something, she says yes, except when that thing is to take a couple hours for herself or to hang out with you. She will bring you food when you are sick or a generator when your power goes out but there is no space in her life to just chill. Every night, every weekend, and even her yearly vacation is overscheduled.

We've all been shades of her before, at some level, at some time. I hope if you are there now you will take a moment to read *Present Over Perfect* by Shauna Niequist. My favorite take-home in that brilliant book is to protect your circles. The first inner circle is your immediate family, husband, and kids. The next circle around that one is best friends or extended family, then close friends, and so on. She encourages you to examine everything in your life that threatens the innermost circles. If there is enough time for the outer rims, then give when you can, but they are not your priority. This means saying no. You don't need to be on every food train, or serve on the board of every activity your kids are involved in. It means taking time to sit and talk and be present (without your phone) with the people you love the most. Not constantly planning for what is next. I'll take it one step further; it means making time for the point in the center of those circles—you. Yes, you want your kids to have every opportunity and play every sport, but you also know that at times they just need to be kids. They don't have to be scheduled every night, they can feel (gulp) bored, and they will actually be better because of it.

By stopping and feeling and saying no and cutting out the busy, you are freed up to hear God. He can then let you truly serve. He will tell you to go sit and listen to your best friend, or cuddle for hours with a struggling child or spouse—things you would previously have no time for in this overscheduled life. In our wait we can get impatient. Just as sitting still in your worry and fear can make you uncomfortable, so can being at rest in the unknown. When you stop moving, when the wait becomes questionable, and you don't know where to go, you start to hear things you don't want to deal with. In order to silence the voices that say you are unworthy, inadequate, and destined to fail, you fill your quiet time with activity, when what you really need is rest. You need to hear your Lord through the lies. God has put you in this downtime so that you can rest and listen for Him.

The beach is my happy place. I know it sounds like an Instagram meme and all summer long you roll your eyes at these hash-tagged words that fill your social media feeds, but I am the person who lives this phrase every single day of the year. In fact, I'm currently typing these words with fingers that I can barely feel as I sit on the porch of my in-law's bay cottage covered in no fewer than six layers of clothing on a frigid winter morning. That's devotion to the shore. Water just calms me, it centers me, it's my ultimate pinot noir. The lake, the bay, the ocean, heck, I'd even take a stream. Just water I can see. So even in the dead of winter, I will haul my family (or sometimes just me, though it's hard for me to leave my little people) to the bay house for a needed mind shift. As I come around the corner before I hit the peninsula, the sky opens up and touches the water. The trees fall away and all I see is bay, sand, boats, and a stretch of old beach houses with stories to tell. My stomach drops a little. I catch my breath and warmth envelops me, even on the coldest of winter days. Relief. Exhale. Air gratefully escaping. I didn't even know I was holding my breath; that's how common the practice is in my life. The cottage comes into view and my heart starts to race a little. Excitement. An eagerness to be in that space. This tiny old combination of wood and water has become where I find rest. There's nothing fancy. No one here to make my bed and serve me meals—not entirely true when my father-in-law is there; he is a pretty awesome cook. It's where I equalize.

There are only two bedrooms, barely enough room for our party of five and parents, but big love grows in small houses. There is a dock and a small boat and turtles and crabs and fish for days. Morning here is my favorite. It doesn't matter the time of year; I will always rise early to sit in an Adirondack chair facing the dock and breathe in my coffee and my Lord. No matter what seems to be going on in my life, this place helps to heal. When things get really tough and I want to escape, my mind always goes to an island with perfect weather, sandy beaches, and staff. Yes, I dream of someone catering to my every need and most importantly, cleaning up! But the funny thing is, all I really need is this little corner of the north-east. A different kind of island. Sometimes it's not a five-star resort or exotic destination, it's just the place that touches a part of you that you didn't even know needed nurturing.

This is where I go to recharge. It's not always easy to get away, and so often it sounds much simpler to stay at home than to drive the hour and a half to the bay, but rest is not often found at home. There's too much to clean and to organize and Target won't shop itself. The red-dressed staff there have come to depend on our frequent visits, and I feel guilty when we stay away too long. At the bay house, cell reception comes and goes with the weather, and the closest store with a door is a twenty-minute drive. I'm never compelled to organize closets or clean toilets because the house isn't my responsibility. When my schedule aligns for a twenty-four-hour escape, I make it a priority to pack up whatever child can come along and head to the water. I know I need the rest. This isn't a vacation, it's a pause. Remember, God rested on the seventh day, He didn't vacuum the basement and meal prep for the week. He rested. If you are like me and you struggle with resting at home, then you need to find a place where you can.

I've created a tiny cove in my home that mimics the bay house. It's no bigger than a short hallway, but it's filled with things that make me happy, spark joy, and encourage calm. There are pictures of the beach, a sign that reads, "breathe," my first article in *Sail* Magazine framed on the wall, and an old door turned into a chalkboard scribbled with my favorite bible verses. I have a comfy chair and pillows that read "seas the day," and "living a blessed life." And there is a window to a wooded area and a far-off creek where in the winter, when the trees are bare, I can glimpse the water. My place of rest amidst the chaos. This is where I retreat every morning. I light a candle, read my bible and whisper to the Lord to find me through the cobwebs of concerns in my head.

I feel your resistance. I know a place to escape isn't easy to find. There are seasons where you can't locate the time to pee in solitude, let alone drive to the beach. The only room you have to yourself is the laundry room and it is anything but inspiring. You don't have family members with beach houses or boats or even a blow-up mattress when you come to visit. None of this means you give up. Come on, you are still here reading this, day after day, praying on your knees, begging for some relief from this wait— you are not one to give up. You are a fighter. Fight for your place in the sun, a room, a location, even a deep breath to get you out of your mind for a minute. You can still find your retreat, so don't stop trying. You have a choice. I had to work hard, and I still do, to make the time to leave my to-do list behind and fight for rest. It really is a war sometimes. I self-sabotage in such remarkable ways. As soon as I'm in a position to rest and receive, my brain seems to conjure up something else to worry about. There are times that I will make the drive and set the intention to rest only to find myself a knot of anxiety and fear for the entire weekend. All of this is a practice. None of what we are learning in these pages will be instantly perfected. We give ourselves grace to make a mistake or to fail and then to try again. But you must keep trying. Find your place in the sun. That location where you can exhale and feel okay even if it's just for a moment.

———✳———

Don't Wait:

- *Stop comparing.* The desire to compare and measure against others' timelines will always be present, but like the fear and the anxiety, practice moving away from comparisons. Whether it be in the pages of a magazine or the people you work with, commit to God's timeline, not someone else's.

- *Clear the List.* Examine why you are always busy. What are you running from or trying to mask with an overscheduled life? Choose yourself, your God, your family, and close friends over all else. That's a big group in itself. Serve them first and then feel free to say yes to the things that fall outside that scope. Take out your planner today and figure out what you can cut out and then circle a few days that have nothing. Sweet, simple, empty nothing. Guard those days for you.

- *Find your happy place.* It doesn't have to be on a grand scale. But find a location, a room, a destination that you can go to and get you out of your head. Figure out how you can get there more often. It will take some juggling and saying no to activities and events, but your peace of mind is much more important.

I waited so long for my person to come along. I often wondered if I would ever get married. I wanted so badly to have kids, but I had to wait. My entire future was on hold until this man came into my life and I could move on. One day I started to pray for my husband, that he was having a happy day, even though I hadn't met him yet! (I know I'm weird.) I started to pray for this unknown guy pretty often. Still waiting, just at least doing something! Funny, that year I met the love of my life, my husband. I literally used to pray for him all the time while I waited to meet him. It all seemed to change when I started to curb my anxiety and loneliness and began preparing to meet him instead of waiting to meet him.

—Nellie

24

SERVE

Before I wrote this book, I knew what my next one would be about. I've had it on my heart for years. Service. The next one will be an account of our family serving others. I even picked out a title and structure. That's how real this future part of my life is to me. It's also a slight illness most writers are never fully cured of: we can't stop writing, no matter how hard we try. And *girl*, how I try. If you think writing books sounds fun, think again. I roll my eyes at that comment almost as hard as I do when people say they would like to "one day adopt." Writing books is hard. Adoption is so, so hard. If you can avoid doing them, your life will be much easier. But if you're like me, God wants you deep in both. At any rate, life would be so much simpler if I could stop processing in paragraphs. But alas, writing is my service. And here we are. Yet despite knowing how important this topic is, this chapter on serving others is the last one I'm going to write in this book. Every other idea came easier. And honestly, I've been putting it off. I've been lacking a hook or an anecdote to better help you understand and identify with the importance of service, when the truth is, there doesn't need to be one. This concept is important enough that it doesn't have to be dressed all pretty. It just needs to get out. And therefore, I just need to write it. Really, it has already been written.

Luke 12:35 reads, "Be dressed ready for service and keep your lamps burning." It's not a new concept. It's been written. In the bible. Instructions from our Lord. Be dressed and ready.

At. All. Times.

It doesn't matter what is going on in your life, you are in a position to serve. Not only are you in a position, you are called to serve. We all are. It doesn't need to be grand or even sacrificial, it just needs to be. Every second of every day, you need to be in a place to serve. That sounds a bit overwhelming with all you have going on. I know I've challenged you to sleep more, eat better, find a support group, memorize scripture, and even cut the fat from your schedule. Now, on top of everything I'm asking you to be ready at any given moment to jump in and serve. Well, yes. Yep, I am. Not apologizing. Just giving it to you like it is. And perhaps it should have been the first thing I told you to do to survive this wait, but it's the last and here we are. Deal.

Here's why: you are strong enough. Don't for a second think your circumstances have made it impossible for you to be of service to others. This weight you are carrying and this pain you feel makes you even more equipped to serve others.

In one of my roughest waiting periods, I was literally legally bound to a job that I hated. I had to go to work every day and fake my happiness because lawyers told me to. I wanted nothing more than to be free from this farce. While I had two babies and a husband to support, I was still more willing to be unemployed than to spend another day in a place full of such negativity. During this horrid waiting period, I was at a stop light about to turn onto a busy intersection and my head was spinning. I couldn't find a way out of this hell. Silly me, I still hadn't learned it wasn't my job to find a way out, but to find out where inside I was needed. My prayers were frequent and intense and while I was begging the Lord for mercy, He told me to pull the car over.

I did, because you don't ignore God. Like ever. Let that be the one lesson you learn: when you think you hear God, you probably did, and so you do what He says.

I parked in a crowded strip mall and got out of my car. I took a twenty-dollar bill out of my wallet and I handed it to a homeless man on the street. A couple things worth noting: 1) I had a twenty in my wallet. Never, ever, do I carry cash. I'm super frugal and I count every penny. Cash is hard to trace in software like Quicken and anything I really need can be put on a credit or debit card. Why I had a twenty-dollar bill in my pocket eludes me, but I have enough faith to say it's a God thing; 2) We were broke. Like broke as a joke. Our first adoption, and all its debt, was still just months behind us; I hadn't paid off the hospital bills from our second daughter's birth and my infertility treatments; my husband's business had just gone under, so he didn't have a pay check; and I was literally *begging* to be unemployed. I had started using Depends as overnight diapers on my daughters because they could be purchased with my flexible spending account. That's how closely I was watching every dime. It saved me, maybe, ten bucks a month. But with that, and the edict that we turned off the water while we lathered up to drive down the water bill, we were able to pay for groceries. 3) Southern California was awash in homeless.

This wasn't a random out-of-luck person on the street that was out of place and could be considered special. During that time, in that city, the homeless were everywhere. They were as common as Los Angeles traffic. This man was not a surprise, nor could he be considered a sign.

To stop my car and pull out a twenty-dollar bill and hand it to a stranger who could very well use it to go buy alcohol at the 7-11 behind us was not in my character.

But God said so, so I did.

I handed over that money and I got back into my car and wept.

But hold on, it wasn't why you think. I wept from relief. Giving that bill away was a huge weight off. It was one less dollar, really twenty less, that I was responsible for. God had to fill that void now, and by me pouring out, He was able to fill me up.

Moments after I pulled away from the strip mall, the phone rang, and my world changed. Not only did that one phone call put an end to the torture I was experiencing at work, but it gave me the ticket to the fulfillment of my wildest dreams. It was that quick. God changed my story in a minute. We hear about that through the bible. We hold it up as evidence. We know, logically, that God is powerful enough to make you say, win the lottery, or be discovered at Wawa, or find out you're royalty, but we don't frequently see that in our lives so it's hard to believe it can happen to us.

Maybe you aren't giving enough to receive.

I am not saying that every time you give, your problems will end. But, could they? If it was just one time out of ten, wouldn't you take those odds? Serving others isn't about what you get in return. That sounds selfish and not what our relationship with God is all about. But He does want to bless you abundantly. Like any good daddy He just wants you to be happy, to see you smile and He knows that by giving, you will get that joy. And for such a time as this, that's exactly what I want you to swallow. The more you give, the more you get. Service is the number one way to survive this wait. It's not just about having your wait be over or your prayers answered, it's about how you feel in the waiting period.

Before that phone rang, I felt relief. As I was pulling out my twenty-dollar bill and walking toward a man who looked frankly dangerous and smelled like I shouldn't approach, I felt resistance. I didn't want to do this thing. I had lost my freaking mind! But as soon as I handed it over and let that part of me go, I felt such calm. Girl, I am never calm. Calm isn't even one of the first fifty words someone would use to describe me. I'm like a Boston Terrier puppy, and it's a wonder I don't pee all over the floor when you walk in the room. But at that moment, in that hot, bright, California strip mall, I felt calm in the chaos. And you know why? It's because I was serving someone other than myself. There was no room for me and my problems and my future tripping. In that moment, I was giving of my heart and my head and of the abundance God had blessed me with. My focus was on someone and something far beyond what was happening in my life.

Serve as often as you possibly can. Give of yourself and your resources in ways you hadn't even considered. It doesn't have to be weekly volunteering at a shelter, though if that is on your heart please, oh please, do just that and shine in the lives of others. It could be inviting someone you know is struggling out for coffee, or sending text messages to friends and family you rarely talk to, just asking how they are and how you can pray for them. How about hosting a bible study once a month at your house? Or asking a neighbor if they need help bringing the trash down to the curb? Service can be in everything we do.

My daughter had a pretty serious accident and was in the hospital. I was at the airport with my other two children and felt like I was barely holding it together. This woman stopped me as we were boarding and told me what a good job I was doing with my kids and how she admired me. She barely spoke English, yet she pushed through her fear to share love. That was such a service to me. Then on the plane when I ordered food, the flight attendant waved away my payment and said with a smile, "sometimes we all just need a little support." She served me and my children. You see, it doesn't have to be big. Just showing kindness to strangers can be service. You never know what they are going through at that moment.

Every time I walk up the steps to my job, I repeat, "I enter this place ready to serve." The building I call home five days a week is massive. We're talking multiple football fields, domed roof, and places in the building that, in eight years, I still haven't explored. I've probably only met half the people who work there, and I get lost trying to find an office at least once a week. This place is rife with service potential. Every day I climb the long cement steps and glance up past the big glass doors and imagine a huge angel hovering its wings over the building. It would be an image that could create nightmares if it were anything but an angel of God. I focus on the protection that is coming from my Lord and I set my heart on not receiving from what's inside, but on giving to who is there. In my years there, I have counseled dozens of women through miscarriage and adoption and infertility. Women who only knew me from TV because their positions are so removed from mine, but who had the courage to reach out to me and ask for help because we work in the same building. Had I not been there, had I not so openly shared my story and continue to this day to tell the truth, we would never have met.

Listen, work can be a challenge. Even when you love what you do, and oh how I love what I do, there are times that the other stuff—the managers, the politics, the contracts and scheduling—can make you question if you're really supposed to be in this place. Spiritual warfare is real with a capital R! When the devil sees so much good happening to further the kingdom of the Lord, he is going to send as much pain and suffering as he can that way. I've been ready to jump ship and get the hell out as fast as I can because I have felt the presence of the devil in a big way. But that's when we are called to dig in deeper. That's when I pause an extra beat and pray harder at the front entrance. That's when I repeat my mantra with every step to my desk and actively look around me for those that are hurting or need help. That's when it's so vitally important to be a soldier for the Lord, a beacon of good. That's when you need to serve as hard as you possibly can.

Service can mean something different for all of us. For me it has a lot to do with finances. I'm still trying to figure out where my dysfunctional relationship with money came from. I was raised for a time by a single mom, but she never let on that we were struggling financially. Then in my teen years, I would have considered us well off. While I was taught early on how to balance a checkbook and the importance of saving, I really never felt we were lacking. We had a great house, the clothes and toys I wanted, vacations every year, and Christmas was nothing short of decadent.

Yet somehow decades later in my own home and marriage I am constantly living in a place of lack. Looking in, you would think I had everything I could ever need, and honestly, I do, but I am constantly stressed about finances. Maybe it comes from having lost so much to adoptions and infertility. It could be the scariness of unemployment that has come numerous times to my family. But you would think having survived tremendous financial devastations would only make me more secure in the Lord's provision. Oh yeah, you would think. Whatever the reason—and be sure, I am deep in therapy to try to figure this one out—for me, money is a roadblock to peace. When I am deep in a waiting period and full of fear and anxiety, my service often needs to be financial. Tithing is line one on the budget, but there are times when I'm so stuck that I honestly need to give more. Like I did with that homeless man in California. Giving it away gave me one less thing to worry about. That act was more than serving him, it also served me.

We are wired for kindness. We just have to recognize that desire in ourselves to help others and then give it as much light as possible so it will grow. Service, giving, and selflessness have always been a part of my life, but not necessarily as much a focus as they are now. It's not that I haven't helped out or given back but I didn't make service a goal. I did it as a part of a checklist. Grocery store, check. Make the bed, check. Volunteer, check! When serving others became a part of my everyday life as opposed to something I had to get done, I began to yearn for more opportunities to help, and then started to recognize that same quality in others around me. What a happier way to live. To see the good in others. There is a whole world full of servants. People like you and me who recognize their purpose is to help. For me it is writing and speaking and sharing difficult stories and, most importantly, being a place where others can feel safe telling theirs. Your job in this waiting period is to figure out what it is for you.

———————✢———————

Don't Wait: discover your purpose in the service realm. How are you called? The best way to develop your gift is to just start doing. Here are a few ways you can start:

- Walk up to a stranger and ask them how you can pray for them.
- Tithe.
- Make a meal for a friend or neighbor.
- Offer to watch the children of someone who you know needs help.
- Google "volunteer" in your city and be amazed at the places that need you.
- Work one day a month at church.
- Hold the door open for five people in a row, and smile and say have a great day.
- Stop and give to a homeless person. Let God decide what they do with that money, that part is not your concern.
- Be the one who does the dishes even if it's not your turn, ditto for any other chore that isn't usually assigned to you.
- Invite someone to coffee or breakfast and let them talk.
- Start a text chain with a group of women who need encouraging, and then be the one who constantly gives praise.

———————✧———————

My mom got sick when I was a teenager, my dad wasn't around, and my grandma helped raise me and my two younger brothers. When she got ill, I didn't think I was going to survive. But God showed me what strength was in the hallways of her nursing home. I learned how to be a caregiver and watched what other families were going through in these facilities and how we all shared the same goal. It was waiting for our loved ones to get healthy enough to go home. Waiting for them to recover so we can move forward to our goals. Never taking life for granted and being thankful for what I had.

—Sandra

25

GREATNESS IS COMING

On my thirty-first birthday, I got a tattoo. That was completely out of character for me. I am averse to pain, and I am a wimp. Paying someone to stick me with a needle repeatedly sounds like the dumbest thing in the world. But I kept thinking about the footnote on this verse I had read in the book of Revelations, and the thought wouldn't leave my mind. It was a positive thought at a time when those were rare. We were nearly three years into the darkness of infertility, and I had spent month after month treating my body like a temple to prepare it for a child, but it wasn't working, and I was done. Angry, disappointed, let down, and done. I wanted to be reminded that I was strong and protected and beautiful, despite how I felt on the inside. So, on my thirty-first birthday, when I had fully planned to be chasing after a toddler, I instead acted like a teenager and got myself a tattoo. I was scared, but so excited, and even after the artist started, I felt happy. I had been pushing the thought away for so long, but the fear was gone when I decided to act.

The tricky part here is that as a girl of God, I'm pretty sure there is somewhere in the bible that it says *don't get a tattoo*—the whole your body is a temple thing. But I had already been abusing my body for so long while trying to get pregnant and I reasoned it was a passage from the bible, so I gave myself a little grace. I walked in the door, held my husband's hand, and got a permanent reminder of a temporary feeling.

If you ever watch me speak you know I like to encourage you to "lean into fear." I truly believe that there can be no growth in your life unless you do the things that scare you. I'm not saying quit your job tomorrow and backpack Nepal when you hate walking, or go skydiving next Tuesday (because that terrifies me and there is no way I'm jumping out of an airplane and I'm pretty sure my life will still be full, thank you very much). I'm talking about the little things like starting a health journey or giving that girl at work a glimpse of your own story because you know she needs to feel like she's not alone. Or like me, getting an itty-bitty baby tattoo when needles freak you out! It's the things that have always gnawed at you, that passion, the dreams, that of which you never speak because it's too scary to think you could actually do it.

So much of what I have moved through in my life has been a result of my choice to take risks. You have read that in this book over and over. I didn't have to decide to adopt, then, *sweet Jesus,* do it again. I didn't have to go through infertility treatments or move seven times in ten years, following my career. No one forced me to write a book, and then another. I could have kept my past to myself and never shared my story. This life I have is because I stayed close to my heart and my Lord and went where He led me. Most of these decisions have brought pain. Yeah, that's a ringing endorsement for risk taking I know, but it's true because each one hasn't been without heartache or anxiety at some point. Choosing to play it safe and isolate could have led to a much more peaceful life in the short term, but that's not what the Lord chose for me, or the three beautiful humans those risks I took produced. There have been scars along the way, but my scars are awesome. The pieces of me I'll never get back but also the places where I gained everything that I am now. We all have them. We can see them as ugly and sad or we can look at them and remember them as a time of growth and faith and grace.

Each scar is a memory of love,
The scar that made me a mother,
The scar that took my own,
The scar where my childhood ended,
The scar that finally healed.

Your scars are gorgeous, my friends. The pain that creates each one is also what makes you beautiful. The time you spend waiting for each chapter of your life to resolve can also produce glorious moments of weeping with gratitude. The hard can be so hard but the good will be beyond the best.

God is in you. And even if (when) you fail in the eyes of the world, or when you get let down by this life, you will always win in the eyes of our Lord. That is where it matters most. It is the Holy Spirit you hear and feel when you can't stop thinking about making that move or taking that chance. Yes, it can be scary, and wouldn't it be easier to just go with the flow and let the world make your path, but you and I both know that is the last thing our heavenly father wants us to do. We are not of this world. We are of Him. His daughters, His servants, His chosen. He is in us and we will not fall. The ledge can seem so daunting and the stakes so high that it would seem the smart thing would be to back away and take a much easier road; but no one ever said being a Christian was going to be easy. In fact, quite the opposite. Being a Christian can be hard. Seriously hard. But it's worth it. Because in you is the joy of the Lord that no one can take, no matter how bad the outcome.

———————⚓———————

That tattoo I have says *144 Cubits*. Look it up in the book of Revelations. It's the height of the wall around Jerusalem, which for me equates to strength and protection, and it's also the exact dimensions of an angel. I love this tattoo. Every time I see it, it makes me happy and reminds me of my Lord. It is a great conversation starter and a tremendous way to tell other people about Jesus. I know, it's crazy that something so borderline heathen has taught me so much about my heavenly father and allowed me to minister to others. This move I made more than a decade ago was a leap for me, but it has led me to do great things. I was in one of the worst periods of my life when I decided to lean into fear, but it produced one of the best parts of my story. There are times in your life where the best of you will come from the worst.

He is pushing you to greatness and helping you grow, or quite simply: He is just using you to grow up baby Christians and watch them populate His kingdom. Perhaps this is what you are meant to learn in this wait, how to help others. Or how to take a chance, a leap of faith, and see what beauty is on the other side of your fear. Around the corner from what looks like a difficult road is greatness. You just need to get through your trepidation to get there.

My bible study and I greet each other with the phrase "greatness is coming." Our friend Lia introduced us to it one day when she was feeling burdened by the weight of so much hardship. She lay her upper body on the big table we were gathered around then rotated her torso and head to the heavens and proclaimed, "greatness is coming Lord!" Even as she was on the proverbial floor, beaten down by all that life could throw at her at that moment, she knew her daddy had incredible plans for her and was going to help her rise from the ashes.

Try it. No matter how low you feel, look up, and insist greatness is on the way. You have learned so much and grown in these pages. You now have the tools to get through this wait and to face the next with power. When the sky seems to be falling, scream it even louder and with more conviction because child, greatness *is* coming.

MEMORIZATION

These are some of my favorite memory verses and phrases. This is a calming tool. Take one at a time and work on repeating until it's easily recalled. I've organized them based on theme. I hope this helps you as much as it has me.

HOPE

Hope for what you do not see.

"Hope for what you do not have, eagerly wait for it with patience." Romans 8:25 (NIV)

"Let your mercy rest on us, O Lord, since we wait with hope for you." Psalm 33:22 (God's Word Translation)

"I will always have hope; I will praise you more and more" Psalm 71:14 (NIV)

For I know the plans I have for you," declares the Lord, "plans for you to prosper, and not to harm you, plans to give you hope and a future. Then you will call on me and come and pray to me, and I will listen to you. You will seek me and find me when you seek me with all your heart. Jer. 29:11–13 (NIV)

FAITH

Speak up, rise up, show up.

"...I will show you my faith by my works." James 2:18 (NIV)

"Watch, stand fast in the faith, be brave, be strong."
1 Corinthians 16:13 (NKJV)

"I am the Lord; I will accomplish it quickly in its time."
Isaiah 60:22 (CSB)

"Keep yourself in the love of God waiting for his mercy."
Jude 1:21 (ESV)

"Surely goodness and mercy shall follow me all the days of my life and I will dwell in the house of the Lord forever." Psalm 23:6 (ESV)

"...continue in the faith, grounded and steadfast, do not move away from the hope of the gospel." Colossians 1:23 (NKJV)

PEACE

With you there is peace.

Greatness is coming.

"You will keep in perfect peace the mind [that is] dependent [on You], for it is trusting in You." Isaiah 26:3 (CSB)

"Yet the Lord longs to be gracious to you; therefore, he will rise up to show you compassion. For the Lord is a God of justice. Blessed are all who wait for him." Isaiah 30:18 (NIV)

"God is in her she will not fall; God will help her at the break of day." Psalms 46:5–6 (NIV)

"Be dressed ready for service and keep your lamps burning." Luke 12:35 (NIV)

"…I have learned to be content no matter the circumstances, I know what it is to be in need, and I know what it is to have plenty. I have learned the secret to being content in every situation. I can do all things through Him who gives me strength." Phil 4:11–13 (NIV)

"I walk in the Lord's presence as I live here on earth!" Psalm 116:9 (New Living Translation)

FEAR

Faith over fear.

Freedom is on the other side of fear.

"Fear produces wisdom when you walk through it."
Year, J.R. Mahon

"Don't be afraid of them, for the Lord your God will fight for you."
Deuteronomy 3:22 (Good News Bible)

"The Lord is the strength of my life; of whom shall I be afraid?"
Psalm 27:1 (NKJV)

"God is our refuge and our strength an ever-present help in trouble. Therefore, we will not fear." Psalm 46:1–2 (KJV)

"Peace I leave you; my peace I give you. I do not give you as the world gives you, do not let your heart be troubled do not be afraid."
John 14:27 (NIV)

"And we know that all things work together for good to those who love God, to those who are called according to His purpose."
Romans 8:28 (NIV)

"God Doesn't promise to save us from the flames but he has promised to be with us as we walk through the fire." Isaiah 43:2 (She Reads Truth Bible)

"There is no fear in love, perfect love drives out fear."
1 John 4:18 (NIV)

WORRY

"Therefore, the Lord is waiting to show you mercy, and is rising up to show you compassion, for the Lord is a just God. All who wait patiently for Him are happy." Isaiah 30:18 (HCSB)

"When my heart is overwhelmed; Lead me to the rock that is higher than I." Psalm 61:2 (NKJV)

"Keep your voice from weeping and your eyes from tears, for the reward for your work will come... There is hope for your future..." Jer. 31:16,17 (CSB)

"...none of the good promises the Lord your God made to you has failed. Everything was fulfilled for you; not one promise has failed." Joshua 23:14 (CSB)

PRAYER

Today, help me live today.

"Listen to your servant's prayer and petition oh Lord my God, so you may hear my prayer and my petition that your servant prays before you today." 2 Chronicles 6:19 (CSB)

"May the words of my mouth and the mediation of my heart be acceptable to you, Lord my rock and my redeemer." Psalm 19:14 (NIV)

"...live a life worthy of the calling you have received." Eph. 4:1 (NIV)

"Since the first day that you set your mind to gain understanding and to humble yourself before your God, your words were heard." Daniel 10:12 (NIV)

"My soul, wait in silence for God alone, for my expectation is from him. He alone is my rock and my salvation, my fortress. I will not be shaken." Psalm 62:6–7 (WEB)

JOY

Joy is a choice.

"The blessing of loss is having experienced great joy."
Year, J.R. Mahon

"Therefore, my heart is glad, and my glory rejoices. My flesh will rest in hope. In your presence is fullness of joy, at your right hand are pleasures forever more." Psalm 16: 9–11 (NKJV)

"I trust in the mercy of God forever and ever, I will praise you forever because you have done it and in the presence of your saints, I will wait on your name, for it is good." Psalm 52:8–9 (NKJV)

"In quietness and confidence shall be your strength."
Isaiah 30:15 (NKJV)

"Many, Lord my God, are the wonders you have done, the things you planned for us. None can compare with you; were I to speak and tell of your deeds, they would be too many to declare." Psalm 40:5 (NIV)

"Praise be to the God and Father of our Lord Jesus Christ, the Father of compassion and the God of all comfort, who comforts us in all our troubles, so that we can comfort those in any trouble with the comfort we ourselves receive from God." 2 Corinthians 1:3–4 (NIV)

"I will turn their mourning into gladness; I will give them comfort and joy instead of sorrow." Jer. 31:13 (NIV)

GRATITUDE

"Heavy things make us stronger."
Susie Larson

THE INSPIRERS:

The Epcot Moms and the Nashville girls for pushing me, taking pictures, wearing tutus and sleeping in bunk beds. Ami for taking my kids and giving me time to create and believing in me perhaps more than anyone else. Melissa for meeting me at my lowest points and showing me pockets of happy. Corie and Brian for always bringing me Jesus. Lia, and all the prayer group girls that have taught me greatness is coming.

THE BRAVE:

Xiomara. Jessica. Vidal.

THE DREAM TEAM:

Dad, the amazing Dr. Lindquist, for being the best proofreader ever and letting me tell your story too, I couldn't have done this without you. Scott for a perfect picture. Maria for giving me confidence and having an anniversary date I'll never forget. Maddie, Allie, Devon, and Patrick for finding me and leading me. Maggie for making this all come together.

The Support System:

Gigi, Dude and Jake, my Delaware dream team. Unknowingly, you all gave me the opportunity to create and serve by caring for and feeding the grandkids while I sat on your beautiful porches.

J.R. Mahon, for reminding me to always wear clothes and get your name right, oh, and saving me, that part too.

THE INNER CIRCLE:

Richelle and Rachel the family I will always choose.

Mame, for always showing me Jesus even when I didn't understand how important He was.

Grace, Georgia, Ben. No words. Just love. A mom that shares it all won't always be easy, but worth it. Your stories help so many, little ones.

Dan. There is no one I'd rather wait with than you. Thank you for supporting every dream and working so hard at making them your own.

My mom. Oh, you above all would understand this need I have to write, and I have to believe you would be proud.

REFERENCES

CHAPTER 2

Stein, Gertrude (1937.) *Everybody's Autobiography.* Virago. Page 298

Niequist, Shauna (2016.) *Present Over Perfect: Leaving Behind Frantic for a Simpler, More Soulful Way of Living.* Zondervan.

CHAPTER 7

Bhandari, Smitha MD (2018.) Retrieved from "Exercise and Depression." Retrieved from https://www.webmd.com/depression/guide/exercise-depression#1

CHAPTER 8

"What do the healthiest people in the world have in common." www.Cbhs.au, 28, March 2018, https://www.cbhs.com.au/health-well-being-blog/blog-article/2018/03/28/what-do-the-healthiest-people-in-the-world-have-in-common

Buettner, Dan (2008.) *The Blue Zone: Lessons for Living Longer From the People Who've Lived the Longest.* National Geographic Books.

CHAPTER 19

Mahon, J.R (2018.) *Year.* Jr@jrmahon.com www.jrmahon.com 619.964.0337

CHAPTER 21

Lindquist, Kerstin (2017.) *5 Months Apart: A Story of Infertility, Faith and Grace.* Elk Lake.

ABOUT THE AUTHOR

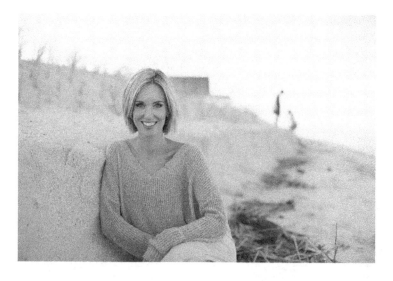

K erstin Lindquist is the author of *5 Months Apart: A Story of Infertility, Faith, and Grace.* She is a four-time Emmy award-winning journalist and recognizable TV host. Her articles on family, fitness, and faith can be seen monthly in various publications from *Vibrant Life Magazine* to *Sail Magazine* and have been featured on *The Today Show.* The confessional nature of her writing and public speaking and the intensely personal stories she shares resonate deeply with her fans. Kerstin lives with her husband and three children in West Chester, Pennsylvania. They spend their free time in warm climates—preferably with sand.